Social Aspects of HIV

Since the start of the epidemic, HIV and AIDS have fired the imaginations of social as well as medical and public health scientists. This innovative series of books offers a setting in which to publish the very best of social scientific thinking and research. The Social Aspects of HIV series of books offers readers authoritative introductions and overviews, together with summaries of enduring and cutting edge concerns. The series is international and multidisciplinary in focus, including contributions from psychology, sociology, anthropology, education, economic, political and social theory, and international development. Individual volumes offer scholarly overviews of key topics and concerns but also address 'big issues' relevant to HIV prevention, treatment and care. Sexual and drug-related practices; adherence; disclosure; and stigma and discrimination are among topics focused upon, alongside broader cultural, political and social responses to the epidemic, including globalisation and internationalisation. The political economy of AIDS, links to broader questions of sexual health and rights, and the progressive biomedicalisation of the response, will also be among key issues examined.The series will appeal to those working in public health, health psychology, medical sociology, medical anthropology, health promotion, social work and international development. Individual volumes will be relevant to students, teachers, researchers and practitioners within each of these disciplines as well as program developers and managers working across a variety of contexts.

More information about this series at http://www.springer.com/series/11922

Robert Lorway

AIDS Activism, Science and Community Across Three Continents

Springer

Robert Lorway
Centre for Global Public Health, the Max
Rady Faculty of Health Sciences
University of Manitoba
Winnipeg, MB, Canada

ISSN 2509-6559 ISSN 2509-6567 (electronic)
Social Aspects of HIV
ISBN 978-3-319-42197-1 ISBN 978-3-319-42199-5 (eBook)
DOI 10.1007/978-3-319-42199-5

Library of Congress Control Number: 2016950717

Printed on acid-free paper

This Springer imprint is published by Springer Nature
The registered company is Springer International Publishing AG Switzerland

Acknowledgements

This book could not have been written without the generosity of numerous individuals. First, I must thank the many activists and community health workers doing activist work who were willing to take the time to teach me about their world, their struggles and their hopes for greater social justice. Over the past 23 years, there are too many such people to mention by name. However, certain activists stand out as having most powerfully transformed my thinking and research pursuits: Wilson Hodder, Jane Allen, Charles Gillis, Bhagya Lakshmi, Prathima Ramaya, Akram Pasha, Jinu Jinendra, Peter Busse and John Mathenge.

I also owe a debt of gratitude to a number of academic colleagues and health scientists over the years who have influenced my thinking around the issues discussed in this book: Lisa Avery, Marissa Becker, Kirsten Bell, Nicole Berry, James Blanchard, Janette Bradley, Sean Brotherton, Fabian Cataldo, Susan Erikson, Denielle Elliot, Elsa Fan, Susan Frohlich, Janice Graham, Ian Harper, Shamshad Khan, Karina Kielman, Deborah McPhail, Lyle McKinnon, Sam Migliore, Michael Montoya, Stephen Moses, Maureen Murney, Kristin Peterson, Stacy Pigg, Peter Redfield, Noelle Sullivan and James Waldram. I was very fortunate to have had the chance to learn from and interact with the very special thinker and being, Vinh-Kim Nguyen. His support and wisdom have meant a great deal to me over the years. Much gratitude is owed to Dr. Sushena Reza-Paul. Her tireless commitment as a physician and health scientist to the communities of sex workers is a constant source of inspiration to me. I am also grateful to have had the chance to work with graduate students who offered compelling questions that influenced the kinds of problems I explore in this book. They include Claudyne Chevrier, Sumit Dutta, Anthony Huynh, Lisa Lazarus, Paula di Migliardi, and Elsabé du Plessis.

Gratitude is owed to the editors and staff of Springer, especially Evelien Bakker and Bernadette Deelen-Mans. I couldn't be more grateful to the distinguished series editors, Peter Aggleton and Richard Parker, for their generous support and patience during the writing process. I am deeply honoured that they approached me with the possibility of contributing to this series.

Considerable thanks is owed to the Canadian Institutes of Health Research (CIHR) and the Social Science and Humanities Research Council of Canada

(SSHRC) Insight Grant Program for their generous funding support, which enabled me to complete various components of the research discussed in this book.

I am also much indebted to my family—my partner Roger, my mother Celia, my sisters Norah and Verne and my brother Charles—for supporting my research pursuits over the years.

Contents

List of Figures

Introduction

Early in the HIV epidemic—amid moral panic, scientific uncertainty and delayed and woefully inadequate government leadership—communities of people living with and directly affected by HIV and AIDS rose to become a powerful force at the forefront of prevention responses, particularly in Euro-American nation-states. "The crisis in biomedicine" in the early years, in part, created the conditions of possibility for grassroots activism and community health initiatives to unfurl and take hold, feeding out from and into an emerging militancy that unleashed visible shows of civil disobedience (Gould 2009). In the absence of a cure or effective treatment, *uncertainty* itself provided fertile ground for AIDS activists to stage protests and lay claim to the legitimacy of their own practical strategies to respond to the epidemic. As the number of experimental HIV treatments grew in the early 1990s, AIDS activism further challenged scientists and on their own territory. For instance, an "impure science" (Epstein 1996) arose in North America in the early 1990s as treatment activists—particularly those based in larger urban centres who possessed considerable intellectual capital and strong alliances with health professionals—began to directly influence the design and execution of clinical trials, forcing their way on regulatory boards, reviewing ethical procedures and pushing access to experimental drugs, on compassionate grounds, for people who had run out of treatment options.

In the late 1990s, following the release of more effective medications, AIDS activism "went global" with transnational networks igniting HIV treatment protests across the world, culminating in the creation of universal access programmes in low- and middle-income countries. Famously, South Africa's Treatment Action Campaign (TAC), which forged influential international alliances, successfully challenged pharmaceutical corporations and, with the political backing of Nelson Mandela, exposed the pharmaceutical industry as enacting a "medical apartheid" (Mbali 2013). In the end, TAC forced drug companies to lower their prices and the South African government to provide affordable access to life-saving medical substances. In another high-profile global demonstration, activists staged a protest at the July 2004 15th International AIDS Society conference in Bangkok, Thailand, an event that brought enormous news media attention to the ethical issues surrounding tenofovir trials running, in the early stage, in Cambodia. The protests of sex workers in fact drove the early shutdown of tenofovir trials based in Phnom Penh. These demonstrations made trial scientists reckon with both the ethical concerns of affected communities and with the influence of transnational activist alliances.

A common thread that runs through these important moments in the history of AIDS activism is the politicization of HIV science, exposing scientific enterprises as being subject to professional and market-oriented interests and nationalistic political agendas. At the same time, the perspectives and tactics of activists were profoundly transformed by the new hierarchies of knowledge that arrived with the release of scientific findings, technologies and health service delivery techniques. As some activists took up various scientific frames of reference to assert their political legitimacy, the "scientization of politics," to borrow Steven Epstein's words, transformed the very ground on which some factions of AIDS activists imagined politics and enacted political dissent. Indeed, "AIDS activism," from the very earliest years, has co-evolved with the development and diffusion of scientific knowledge, and it has lodged some of its sharpest dissenting political perspectives in close proximity to the ideological and material locations of scientific knowledge production.

Successive developments and refinements in HIV biomedical science over the past couple of decades have led us into an era we might consider as the abatement of the biomedical crisis and the diminishment of uncertainty. These developments include highly active anti retroviral therapy (HAART) in late 1995 (with the release of the findings on ritonavir); nevirapine to prevent mother-to-child transmission; medical male circumcision, to reduce HIV infection from women to men; the moderately efficacious phase III RV144 HIV vaccine Thai trial in 2009; treatment as prevention (TasP), building on the use of HAART to prevent mother-to-child HIV transmission; and, most recently, PrEP, with its preventive effects demonstrated in a number of clinical and demonstration trials. These technologies not only hold important implications for the treatment and prevention of people living with HIV; such scientific advances also have, according to Eric Mykhalovskiy and Marsha Rosengarten (2009), "secured the credibility of the biomedical management of HIV," suggesting that the global response has increasingly migrated out of the hands of community-based agencies and towards the custody of clinical, epidemiological and managerial scientific experts. "Re-medicalizing" the HIV epidemic (Nguyen et al. 2011) has indeed given rise to highly technocratic interventions that advance particular global imaginaries of sociopolitical order and rationality while, arguably, submerging the local interests related to human rights and other social justice perspectives.

This technocratic turn is especially embodied in the reigning paradigm governing HIV responses globally—that is, implementation science (IS), an intervention framework that aims to integrate "research findings and evidence-based interventions into healthcare policy and practice" (Schackman 2010). The steady rise in acceptance of IS has indeed intensified the formalization of "the knowledge that counts" to HIV funders and policy makers, a tendency manifest in the almost unquestioning legitimacy of quantitatively oriented knowledge. It is now conventionally assumed in international HIV policy circles that quantitative indicators (along with biological verifications) are best able to define HIV health-related problems, because they measure health outcomes and track accountability to funders. In practice, IS, and the quest for quantitative evidence, has led to the intensification of surveillance of communities, particularly those who are deemed to be "most at risk", "vulnerable" or "key populations," giving rise to enumerative regimes that serve as a testament to the primacy of numbers in governing the response. The quantitative leanings of IS are, perhaps, unsurprising when one considers the fact that IS shares a genealogy with (1) operations research, which employs statistical modelling in attempt to maximize decision making; (2) industrial engineering, also mathematically inclined in its approach to improving efficiency in large and complex systems and processes; and (3) managerial science, which emphasizes costing and quality control (Schackman 2010).[1]

Together, the abatement of the biomedical crisis and the technocratic turn has prompted some scholars to speculate on the end or demise of AIDS activism.[2] *AIDS Activism, Science and Community* responds to this issue in two ways: first by carefully illustrating how activism transforms over time as it becomes entangled in various forms of biomedical, epidemiological and managerial science; secondly, I zoom in on the various social dynamics of collaborations and networks—be they voluntary, uneven, strategic and even coercive—that bring about community activist entanglements with expert forms of knowledge. In this book, AIDS activism follows its own various evolutions as people highly affected by the HIV epidemic engage with intervention programmes initiated by government, humanitarian and academic entities and the host of policy directives and funding conditionalities that seek to govern their participation. What will become evident to the reader is how AIDS activism is not only taking on new forms but, in the era of technocratic and biomedically oriented responses, the contributions of AIDS activism continue to be extremely relevant and important for highlighting social justice concerns.

At the same time, AIDS activism not only transforms and re-emerges within changing scientific and policy conditions, but it also becomes something that can be harnessed when it gets invoked and instrumentalized in interventions. Indeed "community mobilization" is heavily emphasized and even valorized in many contemporary global HIV policy discourses, often under the guise of meeting the principles of the greater/meaningful involvement of people living with HIV and AIDS (GIPA/MIPA). I would argue that approaches to community outreach, empowerment, advocacy and human rights are increasingly being made to serve the interests of clinical, epidemiological and market-oriented scientific experts. These unequal

[1] Newer policy frameworks bandied about in global public health arenas these days, such as programme science, do recognize the central importance of community engagement, but, nevertheless, like implementation science, these frameworks are firmly entrenched in evidence-based public health reasoning that tend to favour the use of advanced mathematical techniques to improve decision making.

[2] Eileen Moyer raised the important question regarding "the end of HIV activism" at the Association for the Social Sciences and Humanities in HIV annual meetings in July 2015. This question is also posed in her abstract which can be found at http://www.aidsimpact.com/2015/Academics/DraftProgramme/abstract/?id=3483.

power arrangements are abetted by neoliberal regimes that have spurred the professionalization and corporatization of AIDS activism, aligning with wider shifts in health policy—such as the move away from community "health promotion" in the 1980s and early 1990s to a pre-occupation with "population health" and "evidence-based" health service delivery in the late 1990s and continuing today.

Grappling with the social, political and concrete health implications of this current moment in the global response to HIV, in this book, I re-create a series of medical anthropological expeditions I conducted across time and space—in Canada, India and Kenya—critically examining various complex entanglements between "cultures of science" and community activism while highlighting the stakes from the perspective of those most affected by the epidemic, especially people using and injecting drugs, female, transgender and male sex workers and gay, bisexual and other men who have sex with men. In the pages that follow, I depict some of the mutual constitutions of (and tensions between) activism and HIV science by drawing upon the findings from an array of community research projects conducted over a 22-year period. I situate "community-based research," which serves as a leitmotif that ties together the seemingly diverse time periods and geographies, within socio-cultural, geopolitical and HIV scientific-historical contexts. Unveiled as a complex site of social connection and struggle, this methodological focus offers an intimate view into the changing political landscapes of AIDS activism and expert knowledge. At the same time, "community-based research" (and its many variants) is exposed as a highly effective instrument that can readily articulate with medicalization and technocratic approaches. The growing expectation for affected communities themselves to produce "sound evidence" to legitimize their advocacy projects and political goals is interrogated throughout the book in relation to its concomitant effects on AIDS activism more generally.

At a moment when "community participation" is increasingly being conscripted into the domain of "global health," I call for the planners and implementers of biomedically oriented HIV research and interventions to more meaningfully engage with communities in ways that de-monopolize decision making—as a matter of ethics and improved scientific practice. But where does activism figure into the possibility of more democratized collaborations between scientists, policy makers and affected communities?

Affective Networks

> As revolutionaries, we always exist in many dimensions, in the passage that is revolutionary, not the final arrival at a new rhythm. And yet, activism is not itself that passage of rhythms; rather, it is a temporary sub-rhythm of denunciation, wounding the first rhythm, from which it carves out a becoming into new territories. (Svirsky 2010)

Instead of delving into a series of iconic struggles that have garnered enormous international media attention over the past three decades or attempting to reconstruct any kind of exhaustive or unified history of how AIDS activism has unleashed waves of dissent throughout the world, this book portrays the more localized, intimate and affective connections that form, dissolve, inflame or tear apart as people gather around projects of social change and confront the possibilities and problems that new scientific knowledge and technologies pose. Emphasizing the more ordinary social textures that undergird everyday projects of defiance (see also Martin et al. 2007), HIV activism, in its multiple embroilments with science, appears as a moving towards change through an opening up of the body to the possibility of affecting others (Gould 2010), while, at the same time, allowing the body to give way to becoming affected by others, including those that express dire opposition. Attention to this kind of circuitous social process—one that "doubles back, increasing its original intensity" (Hemmings 2005:552)—portrays activism as more than defiance that stubbornly stands *against* scientific or technocratic domination, but as a "temporary sub-rhythm of denunciation," borrowing Svirsky's words above, one that begins to alter scientific epistemologies and applications, eventually entwining its dissonant rhythms with science, without ever fully becoming disciplined, subsumed or fully resolved by it. More than defining activism, then, I represent some of the complex everyday makings of the *affective networks* that not only create and re-create the conditions of possibility for activism (also see Dave 2012) but also allow their influence to reach well beyond the collectives of people who identify as being activists or doing activist work.[3] Let me provide an example of how these affective networks might be animated.

During a tea break of a recent HIV-related community research training session I coordinated in August of 2015 with members of a local sex worker and sexual rights CBOs in Abuja, Nigeria, a prominent and outspoken sex work and HIV activist approached me. As a member of the global Network of Sex Work Projects (NSWP), she maintained regular contact with her fellow sex workers across the globe via social media and through periodic international conferences and meetings she attended. She said to me, "You knew Damien—right?"

I nodded, as I had known him well, having worked closely with him over a 3-year period on a community research project in Nairobi, Kenya. I had just received word that he had died of an AIDS-related illness. She then proceeded to hold out her cell phone, displaying a picture of Damien's closed casket, his smiling photo affixed on the top. The casket was suspended above the burial plot into which the body would be lowered as part of the burial ceremony that was taking place. I could see that quite a number of sex workers and their allies, including a clinician I recognized from Kenya and an American researcher, were communicating in real time as the burial ceremony unfolded.

A few others from the workshop gathered around while they continued to display the picture, with the pinging of feedback accumulating on the electronic discussion trail. She then said to all of us, "He was so young. In this day and age, this should

[3] Bobel (2007: 153) draws our attention to the distinction made by some social movement actors between "doing activism" and "being an activist"—the latter being those who "'live the issue,' working very hard and at great personal cost over a long period of time, merit the designation of activist."

not have happened!" A rather halting silence fell over our small group. We gazed at the image of Damien's[4] coffin, at the growing e-discussion trail and at each other, all while remaining quiet. His death was as perplexing as it was tragic. He had died from AIDS, even though he had access to life-saving antiretroviral (ARV) medications. In fact he could not have had better access, since a clinic was based in the CBO office where he regularly volunteered. Having earned the affection of fellow members in his organization, there were many who supported him in adhering to his ARV treatment regime.

A young activist, Damien was only in his late 20s. He had given a revealing public interview that disclosed his HIV status and his profession as a sex worker to a popular online magazine. He had even created a YouTube video detailing how he came to discover that he was gay, explicitly challenging the notion that homosexuality was something imposed by the Western "media or white people," as he put it. Damien always could be counted on to show up for various demonstrations that his organization orchestrated. But the intense discrimination he regularly encountered in the form of police harassment, eviction from his residence, public ridicule over his feminine appearance and gender nonconformity and sexual assaults—all which seemed to fuel his serious alcohol dependency—had "won out" over the wealth of health services and scientific advancement he had at his disposal.

What I want to draw out from this experience relates to the making of affective connections: how the cell phone and the social media website that enabled sex workers to communicate with each other during the funeral, coupled with the image of the Damien's coffin and Fatima's words, opened up *a way for people to react to each other, together, across geographies and social backgrounds*. Yet the moment of showing Damien's casket before it was lowered into the ground yielded more than a series of fleeting affective surges, for Damien was a significant activist who once had participated in the staging of a highly public mass protest in Nairobi in front of the Nigerian High Commission, a demonstration designed to express opposition to homophobic legislation announced in the Nigerian parliament in 2012. Damien also served as a member of the global Network of Sex Work Projects (NSWP), which forcefully announced the rights and interests of sex workers in global HIV policy arenas such as UNAIDS. The point here is that the woman's words—"In this day and age, this should not have happened!"—and the presentation of the cell phone image of the coffin reactivate a sense of these connections and solidarities, stir memories, reaffirm shared histories and political affinities and reignite a sense of togetherness in the continued struggle of stigmatized people with the HIV epidemic, social discrimination and biomedicine. Thus, there is an inherent futurity invoked in her words, a future that has not yet arrived but that powerfully animates these affective networks. In other words, the women's exclamation was a powerful evocation of the work that was still outstanding for AIDS activists and their allies.

What emerges in my analysis in this book is recognition of the important role played by the evocative words and stories that activists tell and retell to each other

[4] All participants' names are pseudonyms.

and to themselves and how the building of affective networks is always on the verge of breaking out into—of becoming—political thinking and action.[5]

Evidentiary Sovereignty

But where do we locate scientists in relation to this affective terrain? The HIV epidemic is somewhat unique as a health problem in the extent to which health scientists and highly affected communities have been brought into close proximity with each other, in the mutual working out and continual refinement of programmes, procedures and approaches— attuning to the contexts and complexities of the lives of highly marginalized or stigmatized people in the shared goal of improving prevention to HIV infection and the delivery of health services. We should, then, not entirely situate HIV scientists and experts outside the reaches of affective networks. Across the three sites in which I have conducted ethnographic research, I found a number of impassioned clinicians, public health specialists, scientists, researchers and even government officials who had become close allies to highly affected communities and deeply affected themselves. Some of these experts even appeared to become welcomed by activists into the definition of "the community." However, in the era of "treatment as prevention" and implementation science, there is also a growing chorus of biomedical and public health experts that questions the importance of "human rights-based approaches" and treats activism as though it were inimical to the aims of "scientific progress" and "technical advancement."[6] With the technocratic turn in the HIV response, what does this spell for the ability of outspoken community activists to affect the intensification of technical authority in policy arenas?

On the one hand, the discourse of "evidence-based decision making" has certainly opened up new territories upon which dissenting views have begun to unfold. For instance, in 2015, the sex worker-run and sex worker-led global Network of Sex Work Projects (NSWP) gathered together the complaints and anxieties of its member organizations by commissioning their own study that documented some of the misuses of a geographic mapping technique used throughout the world in the design, planning and resource allocation of HIV interventions for sex workers and sexual minorities (NSWP 2015). Their report also raised objections around the use of biometrics such as electronic fingerprinting with communities who live under the

[5] My thinking here owes much to feminist geographer Deborah G. Martin and colleagues who note how "localized interactions and may evolve into more formalized, institutional social movements" (Martin et al. 2007: 78). They consider activism "as everyday actions by individuals that foster new social networks or power dynamics. In this sense, we see activism as a precursor to political action that transforms a community, develops a formal organization, or extends in scale to reach social networks beyond the initial embeddedness of the instigating activist."

[6] Nguyen and colleagues (2011: 291) comment on the opening address made by Julio Montaner at the 18th International AIDS conference in which he proclaims the importance of treatment as prevention "over and above the human rights issues."

shadow of criminalization. This report has not only been widely circulated, but its findings have been heard by high-level global health officials and leading epidemiologists. And it has made its way into international forums and conferences where influential policy makers gather. On the other hand, "evidence-based decision making" also displaces and diminishes the affective force of the kinds of narratives that activists tell and retell each other, and it elides and delegitimates the significance of the wealth of local, practical knowledges that have accumulated in HIV community-based organizations over decades, what scholars writing in the participatory research literature often refer to as "community wisdom" (see, e.g., Stevens and Hall 1998, Gehlert and Coleman 2010 and Shalowitz et al. 2009).

As increasingly narrow forms of quantitative knowledge come to rule global HIV decision-making arenas, HIV CBOs have been forced to adapt, often making research and other formalized knowledge production methods that generate "acceptable forms of evidence" their close companion to assert their advocacy concerns, while satisfying accountability to funders in strict, measurable terms. Furthermore, uneven collaborations with clinical researchers have become a necessary mainstay for many sex worker and sexual minority rights CBOs, particularly in low- and middle-income countries. Guided by programme directives, such as the Global Fund to Fight AIDS, Tuberculosis and Malaria (GFATM), President's Emergency Plan for AIDS Relief (PEPFAR), Atlanta Center for Disease Control (CDC), Centers for Disease Control and Prevention (CDC) and the Bill & Melinda Gates Foundation (BMGF), CBO leaders and activists increasingly find their daily work embroiled in enumerative procedures, quantitative indicators, biological-behavioural surveillance and myriad reporting requirements. Of course, taking on these responsibilities becomes necessary to survive the operating costs of keeping CBOs afloat, amid dwindling public, governmental and humanitarian financial assistance (Fan 2014). Sexual and gender minorities and sex workers who live in countries where their specific health concerns are largely ignored in the healthcare system indeed welcome the specialized health services and biomedical resources that come with the medicalization of HIV prevention and care; other important issues that exist outside the biomedical-epidemiological gaze, but which are nevertheless crucial to the health and well-being of affected communities, also fall out of view. In the chapters that follow, my ethnographic depictions reveal some of these overlooked realities.

In thinking about the widening epistemological displacement of community activists and health workers in HIV responses where I have studied, I have continually returned to a number of questions pertaining to the notion of sovereignty. Although defined in a variety of ways by social and political theorists, the cases discussed in this story are guided by an understanding of a mode of rule that I characterize as *the power to decide upon the knowledge "that counts"* in HIV policy-making arenas, what I call evidentiary sovereignty.[7] This definition of sovereignty is

[7] My way of thinking about power, like Rouse and Samsky, shares an obvious affinity with French poststructural thinker Michel Foucault (1980) and the knowledge/power regimes he famously articulated in his writing.

much informed by Joseph Rouse' (1996: 3) discussions of "epistemic sovereignty" which highlights how power is "deployed outside the framework of the state apparatus or class domination" and how sovereignty operates in the relationships between scientific knowledge and politics as an "epistemological problematic."[8] My concept of evidentiary sovereignty also takes inspiration from Samsky (2012): "scientific sovereignty is the power formation that uses industry-supported biomedical innovation to drive state action, and that replaces the state as the primary actor in biopolitical power relations" (317). Much like Samsky's notion, evidentiary sovereignty exists as "a leaderless, difficult to describe coalition of industry, multilateral, and nongovernmental organizations that references health itself as a justification for its power" (317). However, I am more preoccupied with conveying an understanding of the everyday workings of these coalitions—how they puzzle through and decide what constitutes "evidence" or what counts as acceptable knowledge.[9]

My conceptualizing of evidentiary sovereignty (related to decision-making arenas concerned with protecting and enhancing the health of "vulnerable populations") is based upon more than 20 years of empirical work, including experiences and observations made during the myriad meetings, conferences, funding review panels and working groups attended over the past two decades—meetings that brought together diverse groupings of social actors, including government health officials, scientists, healthcare professionals, funders and affected communities. These gatherings often assembled under the banners of "collaboration," "partnering" and "consultations," where competing epistemological claims were posed and where policies affecting those who gain access to life-saving resources (and others from which resources can be withheld) were formed. Although a plurality of epistemologies exert agency in these types of discursive arenas, *sovereignty operates in this practical field of decision making as diverse social actors negotiate and renegotiate particular hierarchies of knowledge*, working them out through contestation and deference, opposition and capitulation. At the same time, we must be mindful of the important role that affective ties and networks play in holding together these discursive formations, which raises a number of important theoretical questions about the very nature of the ground on which emotion, politics and rationality are mutually constituted.[10]

By considering the exercise of evidentiary sovereignty as it unfolds in an assembly of HIV intervention decision-making practices across seemingly disparate geographies and temporalities, I have come to realize that the emergent knowledge

[8] As Healy insists, "'Epistemic sovereignty' thwarts attempts to democratise knowledge and decision-making because the presumption of 'sovereignty' unavoidably marginalises other perspectives and views, embedding the power relations underpinning the status quo" (Healy 2003: 693).

[9] My perspective on sovereignty—as operating in and through quotidian moments of decision making—intersects with the ideas of anthropologist Stacy Piggs's discussion of global health and ethnography (2013) in which she mobilizes the metaphor of "sitting and doing" to portray the nonlinearity of decision making in global health in an effort to call attention to the need for a critical reflexivity around how problems and calls to action are framed in global health.

[10] In other words, attention to the role of affect in the co-evolution of activism and science questions Weber's conceptualization of emotion and reason as firmly oppositional.

hierarchies I have been studying do not configure quite the same way in every location. Although the standardizing effects of global health guidelines and orthodoxies certainly may create parallel problems for CBOs and HIV activists throughout the world, the reigning forms of expertise that undergird such global regulatory regimes cannot be entirely conceptualized as a universalizing force that operates beyond the boundaries of nationalism, as it acts upon various responses.[11] Instead, by attending to *the more particularistic remakings of knowledge hierarchies as they unfold in specific locales,* I characterize the operation of evidentiary sovereignty as pivoting around cultural milieus, historical specificities, national interests and questions concerning the changing conditions of health citizenship.[12]

Writing Engaged Ethnography

As an ethnographer trained in social and cultural anthropology, the story I tell of how forms of HIV activism entangle and co-evolve with scientific and other expert knowledges is based on a combination of fieldwork techniques—observations, note taking, interviewing, audio recording, visual analysis, examination of organizational literatures and archival retrieval and analysis—all of which are rooted in relations of rapport and the idea that data pertaining to social reality is best generated through intensive interactions between "the researcher" and "the researched". Over the past 21 years of ethnography, my engagement in the field of HIV research has shifted tremendously. I began as a graduate student-level researcher based in community activist-run organizations, and, over time, I became an academic working in a medical school-based, global health centre that provides ongoing technical support to large-scale interventions in parts of Asia and Africa. Against the backdrop of HIV scientific advances, my changing positionalities have greatly affected my engagements with activists, scientists and health officials. Moreover, holding these

[11] My thinking takes cues from Didier Fassin's discussion of the obscurity of global health: "rather than being submitted to supranational political determinations and inscribed in an ethical order without boundaries, [the globalization of health] continues to be principally ruled by national interests and state sovereignties, primarily serving local constituencies" (Fassin 2012: 99; also see Anderson 2014:375). Fassin's words echo in Anderson (2014) who questions the larger academic enthusiasm surrounding "global flows" and instead views the travel of science and medicine across national borders through a postcolonial lens. "Historians along the North Atlantic shores," he argues, "are forsaking national narratives for global explanations, preferring transnational agency to situated structure" (Anderson 2014:375).

[12] Colvin and Robbins (2009) assert that "analysts of health citizenship," particularly singling out Nguyen's notion of therapeutic citizenship, "often overestimate the power and reach of global assemblages…to inculcate and produce these new forms of health citizenship." They insist that "the power of biomedicalization, and the forms of therapeutic citizenship that are associated with it, only emerges out of the linking of these global discourses and technical practices with both existential/embodied changes in individuals and the reorganization of social roles and expectations at the local level that (sometimes) accompany global biomedical interventions. And this imbrication of the global and the local is always dynamic, uncertain, and often, an uneasy project" (180).

multiple positionalities has afforded me with an array of vantage points from which to view and experience the complex workings of evidentiary sovereignty in HIV policy decision-making arena.

My earliest ethnographic work began in the eastern Canadian province of Nova Scotia, where my initial research questions closely entwined with my volunteer work, and grew out of concerns shared with me by AIDS activists and people living with HIV and dying from AIDS-related illnesses. Between 1991 and 1999, my research activities were an integral part of the work I was doing with community-based organizations leading responses in the Atlantic Canada region. During this period, I also came to serve as the acting training coordinator for the AIDS coalition of Nova Scotia, when the regular coordinator was on extended sick leave. This meant that I was temporarily given the responsibility of coordinating the STI/HIV anonymous testing clinic in the organization and was tasked with fostering relationships with men in the community who identified as gay and bisexual, so as to connect them to the community friendly sexual health services. In 1998, I was made the research director of ACNS to coordinate a community-based research capacity building project, a Health Canada initiative that later brought me into close contact with a range of influential HIV prevention actors across Canada, including academic researchers, Health Canada representatives and community activists and advocates.

After completing doctoral research among sexual minorities in southern Africa in 2005,[13] my research migrated more explicitly towards the world of public health when I began to pursue a postdoctoral training programme in infectious diseases and global health at the University of Manitoba. I then took up an academic position in health sciences at Simon Fraser University before returning to the University of Manitoba, where I currently make my academic home. Becoming an inhabitant of the world of applied public health practice, I was exposed to large-scale interventions, throughout Asia and Africa, led by multinational teams of health scientists and programme managers. As I came to work alongside public health scientists on some of these interventions, I often came to be seated on what sometimes felt like "the opposite side of the table" from community activists, until I was able to rebuild relations of rapport with them over the coming months and years.

Being situated in a medical school is not an entirely comfortable location to occupy for an anthropologist trained in critical social theory, especially when social scientific epistemologies and perspectives suffer regular institutional devaluations. The academic performance of the few social scientists in my department is regularly compared to faculty in other fields where long-term field work and lengthy theoretical papers are not expected in their respective fields. In many ways, residing in this multidisciplinary location has become an important field site that has greatly attuned my analysis of how sovereignty and expert knowledge production operate through complex social practices, as I regularly witness the ways diverse epistemological posturings play out during committee and faculty meetings.

[13] I discuss the details of this ethnographic work elsewhere (Lorway 2014) focussing more on development work rather than public health projects.

Having made my academic home in a global public health centre, I am regularly expected to "put my anthropology where my mouth is" with respect to ongoing applied global health interventions in Asia and Africa led by the University of Manitoba Centre for Global Public Health faculty. What this means is that when I raise particular conceptual criticisms around global health interventions, I am expected to not only conduct studies to back up my assertions, but I am also expected to make concrete suggestions that will contribute to the amelioration of health struggles. While this latter expectation is not entirely out of step with my own activist leanings, what this has meant for me, at times, is to become uncomfortably entangled and implicated in the very objects of my critique, as I come to share in responsibility for the effects of the very health programmes I study. However, pushing and reworking the disciplinary edges of my training in critical medical anthropology (Singer 2004) has not led me to the conclusion of the impossibility of producing robust and edgy critical insights; instead, I find myself in an entirely different location from which to theorize, a location where critical studies of health continually resist and push beyond the dichotomy of a social science "in" versus the social study "of" public health. (Over time I have come to wonder how anthropologies "of" public health can ever be accomplished without direct immersion and participation *in* the very terrains of applied practice where particular social and political realities are constructed.) Hopefully this book points to the productiveness of the friction that recurs when holding critical and applied health research in tension.

Being based in a medical school also allows me to be immersed in cultures of biomedicine. Unaware that I am not a physician, on almost a regular basis, pharmaceutical companies or other private sector biomedical firms email me to review patient charts and to supply them with data, with an offer of payment. In other words, I regularly get to peek behind the curtain to see how commercial and private interests routinely colour the practice of biomedicine. This has helped me to understand the lack of discomfort and concern expressed by some physician scientists at my institution with respect to the employment of business science to govern health interventions, for market-oriented logics have already imbued their daily practices, such that they appear unremarkable to them. I can recall when Ashok Alexander, former director of the global management firm McKinsey & Company and also former director of the HIV initiative in India known as Avahan, met with our faculty at the Centre for Global Public Health and informed us of his vision for public health. Part of that vision is encapsulated in the following statement he made: "public health is focussed on *supply side* but it needs to focus more on *the demand side*, on *the consumers*—the community." In general, I found Alexander's discussion with us both compelling and concerning. On the one hand, he recognized the critical role of local communities in public health programmes. On the other hand, the deference to management science and marketing ideologies throughout his talk failed to engage any fundamental critique that implicated capitalism in the production of health inequities. Instead, virtuous market forces were imagined to rescue disenfranchised people from ill health.

This example exemplifies a form of irony that is continually restaged in the world of academic health science and in the concrete field of applied practice where I conduct my ethnographic research: health scientists in Canada, India and Kenya regularly trumpet the importance of health equities research, the social determinants of health and the need for attention to the structural inequalities surrounding vulnerable populations; yet any sustained critiques of how global capitalism may actually contribute to the arrangement of health inequities remain curiously absent. This irony forms an important subplot in the story that follows—that is, how myriad marketing interests are often masked behind the supposedly neutral assertions of scientific knowledges, technologies and intervention techniques that get expressed in spaces where decisions are made that profoundly affect the well-being of people living with and vulnerable to HIV.

Winnipeg, MB, Canada Robert Lorway

References

Anderson, W. (2014). Making global health history: The postcolonial worldliness of biomedicine. *Social History of Medicine*. hkt126.

Bobel, C. (2007). 'I'm not an activist, though I've done a lot of it': Doing activism, being activist and the 'perfect standard' in a contemporary movement. *Social Movement Studies, 6*(2), 147–159.

Colvin, C., & Robins, S. (2009). Positive men in hard, neoliberal times: Engendering health citizenship in South Africa. In *Gender and HIV/AIDS: Critical perspectives from the developing world* (pp. 177–190). Farnham: Ashgate Publishing Limited.

Dave, N. N. (2012). *Queer activism in India: A story in the anthropology of ethics*. Durham: Duke University Press.

Epstein, S. (1996). *Impure science: AIDS, activism, and the politics of knowledge* (Vol. 7). Berkeley: University of California Press.

Fan, E. L. (2014). HIV testing as prevention among MSM in China: The business of scaling-up. *Global Public Health, 9*(1–2), 85–97.

Fassin, D. (2012). That obscure object of global health. In *Medical anthropology at the intersections: Histories, activisms, futures* (pp. 95–115). Durham: Duke University Press.

Foucault, M. (1980). *Power/knowledge: Selected interviews and other writings, 1972–1977*. New York: Pantheon.

Global Network of Sex Work Projects (NSWP). (2015). *Mapping and population size estimates of sex workers: Proceed with extreme caution*. http://www.nswp.org/tags/ethical-research.

Gehlert, S., & Coleman, R. (2010). Using community-based participatory research to ameliorate cancer disparities. *Health & Social Work, 35*(4), 302–309.

Gould, D. B. (2009). *Moving politics: Emotion and ACT UP's fight against AIDS*. Chicago: University of Chicago Press.

Gould, D. (2010). On affect and protest. In *Political emotions* (pp. 18–44). New York: Routledge.

Healy, S. (2003). Epistemological pluralism and the 'politics of choice'. *Futures, 35*(7), 689–701.

Hemmings, C. (2005). Invoking affect: Cultural theory and the ontological turn. *Cultural Studies, 19*(5), 548–567.

Lorway, R. (2014). *Namibia's Rainbow Project: Gay rights in an African nation*. Bloomfield: Indiana University Press.

Martin, D. G., Hanson, S., & Fontaine, D. (2007). What counts as activism? The role of individuals in creating change. *Women's Studies Quarterly, 35*(3/4), 78–94.

Mbali, M. (2013). *South African AIDS activism and global health politics*. London: Springer.

Mykhalovskiy, E., & Rosengarten, M. (2009). HIV/AIDS in its third decade: Renewed critique in social and cultural analysis–An introduction. *Social Theory & Health, 7*(3), 187–195.

Nguyen, V. K., O'Malley, J., & Pirkle, C. M. (2011). Remedicalizing an epidemic: From HIV treatment as prevention to HIV treatment is prevention. *AIDS, 25*(11), 1435.

Pigg, S. L. (2013). On sitting and doing: Ethnography as action in global health. *Social Science & Medicine, 99*, 127–134.

Rouse, J. (1996). *Beyond epistemic sovereignty*. Division I Faculty Publications. Paper 37. http://wesscholar.wesleyan.edu/div1facpubs/37.

Samsky, A. (2012). Scientific sovereignty: How international drug donation programs reshape health, disease, and the state. *Cultural Anthropology, 27*(2), 310–332.

Schackman, B. R. (2010). Implementation science for the prevention and treatment of HIV/AIDS. *Journal of Acquired Immune Deficiency Syndromes* (1999), *55*(Suppl 1), S27.

Singer, M. (2004). Critical medical anthropology. In *Encyclopedia of medical anthropology* (pp. 23–30). New York: Springer US.

Shalowitz, M. U., Isacco, A., Barquin, N., Clark-Kauffman, E., Delger, P., Nelson, D., et al. (2009). Community-based participatory research: A review of the literature with strategies for community engagement. *Journal of Developmental and Behavioral Pediatrics, 30*(4), 350–361.

Stevens, P. E., & Hall, J. M. (1998). Participatory action research for sustaining individual and community change: A model of HIV prevention education. *AIDS Education and Prevention, 10*(5), 387.

Svirsky, M. (2010). Defining activism. *Deleuze Studies, 4*(supplement), 163–182.

Part I
Canada: Professionalization

Chapter 1
A Vital Response

Abstract This chapter specifically portrays how a grassroots response to the HIV epidemic began to transform as Health Canada welcomed "the HIV movement" in Nova Scotia into the fold of legitimacy with operational funding, ushered in by the community health promotion discourses that were powerfully re-articulated in 1986. Vivid protests staged by activists indeed exemplified the reigning ideals of community empowerment reiterated in larger Health Canada policy forums at the time. Eventually, a group of mostly HIV positive people and their close allies emerged as the victors in the struggle to lead the local response in Nova Scotia, and accepted government operating funds. However, the once seemingly clear dividing line between AIDS activists and "the oppressor" began to blur as the members of the AIDS Coalition of Nova Scotia became increasingly drawn into the project of governing the response as the activist community submitted to relations of accountability with the federal government funder, Health Canada, and the provincial funder then known as the AIDS Community Action Project. Conversations and interviews conducted with activists that began in 1992 and continued until 1999 reveal how evidence-based program rationalities were becoming firmly entrenched in community practises and ideologies.

Keywords History of HIV and AIDS activism • Discrimination • Canada • Community-based research

AIDS Activism in the capital city of Nova Scotia, Canada, like in many other urban settings across North America in early 1980s, was forged out of the realities of discrimination, delayed and ineffective government leadership, and biomedical inadequacy. People who were sick with AIDS were left to die through intensely discriminatory practises enacted within the very institutions where they sought health care. Reinforcing such exclusionary practises within the health care system, the Canadian government's reticence to engage with HIV and AIDS as an urgent crisis facing particular groups of people intensified their marginality and saw the needs of people dying from AIDS largely ignored in provincial and national government policy, until the long-awaited first national AIDS strategy in 1989. Coupled with a negligent state, a "crisis in biomedicine" ensued over the lack of a cure, effective treatments, or vaccines on the near horizon. In Nova Scotia, the many gay men I came to know through my ties to "the movement" shared their narratives of how

R. Lorway, *AIDS Activism, Science and Community Across Three Continents*, Social Aspects of HIV 1, DOI 10.1007/978-3-319-42199-5_1

they had returned from larger urban centres like Vancouver, Toronto, New York, Los Angeles and Miami "to die at home" in the small maritime island of Cape Breton, where I lived at the time. Some of these men "came out" to their families for the first time as gay men, and they did so while also disclosing a highly stigmatized, terminal illness.

The replaying of this tragedy of discrimination, loss, and death gave rise to radical AIDS activism that this chapter explores. I begin therefore by discussing the productiveness of death in how it galvinized political objectives and bonded together activist communities (also see Murray 2008).[1] In fact, the loss of life during this period nourished a vital, edgy, and subversive response from gay communities, one that unleashed highly visible protests against the state, while strengthening the bonds of social solidarity between activists and their allies. I also portray how a grassroots response to the HIV epidemic, which unfurled into a spirited activism, began to transform as Health Canada welcomed "the HIV movement" into the fold of legitimacy with operational funding, ushered in by the community health promotion discourses that were powerfully re-articulated in 1986 (World Health Organization 1986). Vivid protests staged by activists indeed exemplified the reigning ideals of community empowerment reiterated in larger Health Canada policy forums at the time. Eventually, a group of mostly HIV positive people and their close allies emerged as the victors in the struggle to lead the local response in Nova Scotia, and accepted government operating funds. However, the once seemingly clear dividing line between AIDS activists and "the oppressor" began to blur as the members of the AIDS Coalition of Nova Scotia (ACNS) became increasingly drawn into the project of governing the response as "the HIV movement" submitted to relations of accountability with the federal government funder, Health Canada and the provincial funder then known as the AIDS Community Action Project.

Retracing parts of this local history, I want to focus on my conversations and interviews conducted with activists that began in 1992 and continued until 1999, at which time evidence-based program rationalities were becoming firmly entrenched in community practises and ideologies related to community-based research.

1.1 What Will Become of Us?

In the spring of 1997, program staff and board members of the AIDS Coalition of Nova Scotia (ACNS) called a meeting to discuss an upcoming provincial needs assessment funded by Health Canada's AIDS Community Action Project (ACAP), a study that was expected to engage community AIDS organizations across Nova

[1] This line of thought it informed by Stuart Murray's discussion of thanatopolitics and the uses of death in politics, which focuses on the other side of biopolitical sovereignty pertaining to those who can be "let die" when considered a threat to human security. This contrasts with the more common emphasis in scholarly discourse placed on how techniques of government move to enhance life or "make live."

Scotia. During this meeting, the activist Wilson Hodder and other members of ACNS reiterated the importance of the needs assessment, claiming that is was necessary to reflect on "the uncertainty for the future direction of the HIV movement". How were they to proceed amid dwindling funds from Health Canada, staff cut backs, and new government policies that shifted focus away from community health promotion principles, which emphasized collective action "from below", to a "top-down" population health framework that emphasized a more epidemiological perspective on the health of people most highly affected by HIV and AIDS? Moreover, ACNS had to contend with neoliberal funding reforms that emphasized a more "professionalized" approach to "training" and "partnership building" to expand the role of ACNS and to "mainstream" and "democratize" AIDS so it could be viewed as an illness like any other within the provincial health services landscape. Toward the end of the 1990s, complaints abounded among ACNS staff regarding Health Canada's requirement of increasing reporting requirements, which left them with less time to spend with actual members, delivering supportive health services.

Following the meeting, Wilson Hodder invited me into his office where he continued to lament on the "political malaise" that had begun to set in among members of the HIV movement in Nova Scotia. After digging through a box of files, while continuing to mutter in an irritated tone, he finally handed me a copy of a speech that Vito-Russo once delivered during an Act-up rally in New York and insisted that I somehow include some of the text in the assessment write-up I was contracted to compose for ACNS. Wilson pointed out one passage in particular, which I also highlighted in the eventual assessment report:

> You know, living with AIDS in this country is like living in the twilight zone. Living with AIDS is like living through a war which is happening only for those people who happen to be in the trenches. Every time a shell explodes, you look around and you discover that you've lost more of your friends, but nobody else notices. It isn't happening to them. They're walking the streets as though we weren't living through some sort of nightmare. And only you can hear the screams of the people who are dying and their cries for help. No one else seems to be noticing.
>
> And it's worse than a war, because during a war people are united in a shared experience. This war has not united us, it's divided us. It's separated those of us with AIDS and those of us who fight for people with AIDS from the rest of the population.[2]

Wilson was himself a much admired activist. He spoke out openly about his HIV positive status and the injustices committed against PLWHA in local and national new media. Impressively, he launched (and eventually won) a personal court case in 1995 for same sex benefits after his partner of many years died of AIDS. In his own activism, Wilson drew much inspiration from the AIDS activist group ACT-UP (the AIDS Coalition to Unleash Power) in New York and in a later interview this sentiment was reflected when I asked him how he felt about the changes occurring around AIDS activism in Halifax:

> In those [early] days, it was very much a reactive thing … a politician would say some stupid remark in the press.... AIDS was a media draw at that time … if we said anything

[2] The full speech can be found at http://www.actupny.org/documents/whfight.html

> about AIDS we got media attention … we were AIDS activists … it was "act up"…people chaining themselves to the stock exchange in New York.
>
> One year [in Halifax] we rented a donkey from the valley … to point out the slowness, the "*ass*-inine" policies of the provincial government … and without a permit we paraded through downtown towards the legislature and we stuck condoms on anything protruding around the Nova Scotia legislature (jokingly) … and of course that created a lot of media attention … on the way there we had "die-ins" at the intersections … I think we even flabbergasted the police … they were driving by on one side of the street, we were marching down the other side in the street not on the sidewalk … we were activists then. We have passion now, but we don't have the passion we had then. Then we would just do things. If someone said let's have a demonstration, then we would have a demonstration. We could call and get 50 people in an hour … now I don't think we could get 50 people if we were planning for a month. (Oct. 1998)

Wilson was certainly not alone in his nostalgic laments. A number of the HIV movement organizers I spoke with in Nova Scotia became gravely concerned with what they characterized as the growing political apathy of its members. The political achievement of ACNS in becoming a visible and accepted institution within the provincial health services landscape and the promising developments in treatment options that shifted the framing of HIV as a terminal illness to a chronic manageable condition at the end of 1995 (see Chap. 2), together, seemed to take the wind out of the political sails of the organization. For this reason, the staff and board members of ACNS decided that the needs assessment should not only examine their "current program gaps" for future planning, but they should also assess the pre-existing capacity of the HIV movement by reconstructing a history of the movement itself. It was expected that the production of this history would help revitalize the movement in planning the way forward.

1.2 Come Together!

In 1982 a small group of gay physicians and people living with AIDS and their partners banded together to form the Gay Men's Health Group in Halifax. Based on information they received from the Gay Men's Health Crisis in New York, this group formed without funding after the first few people in Halifax were diagnosed. This loosely organized group had no office but met in each other's living rooms and kitchens to discuss how best to respond to the epidemic facing gay men in Halifax. Some activists I interviewed described this collective as primarily a support group for those who became sick with AIDS. This group did not engage with the media and was largely invisible to the public, although they did hand out educational pamphlets to patrons at a local gay bar known as *Rumours*. Rumblings from the emergent networks of AIDS activist quickly grew around having the word "gay" in the name of the association; and by 1983 the organizers changed it to MACAIDS. Members of MACAIDS actively sought out and met with hospital staff, provided information to public health nurses and some physicians. They tended to focus mostly on health systems reform and community outreach.

In the early mid to 1980s, AIDS activism in North America grew in resistance to a climate of moral panic and human rights violations. Nova Scotia activism in many ways paralleled the movements of larger urban centres such as New York's ACT UP (Stoller 1998). One key event that sparked a more radical arm of the HIV movement in Nova Scotia was the case of Eric Smith which grabbed national and international news headlines in 1986. Eric Smith, from Clarkes Harbour in Shelburne country Nova Scotia was an openly gay elementary teacher who in 1986 was diagnosed as being infected with HTLV-III/lymphadenopathy (HIV).[3] His status was later disclosed to the community in which he lived by his family doctor's receptionist in 1987. As a consequence, he was removed from his teaching position. The Shelbourne county municipal councillors also voted to ban "AIDS infected" people and "homosexuals" from teaching students (Numer 2014: 3; Jones and Sheppard 1989). Such blatant discrimination had a profound effect in further mobilizing AIDS activism in Nova Scotia.

Eventually responding to this event, the provincial government established the Nova Scotia AIDS Taskforce, the formation of which many local activists claimed was an attempt to save face amid their failure to take responsibility for and manage the controversy, as one activist maintains:

> The provincial government was absolutely pathetic in their response to AIDS. They couldn't handle the Eric Smith crisis. The government should have been taken to court and challenged but nobody chose to do that … It was an absolute disgrace and the government chose to do nothing other than form a fucked up commission to do nothing. Of course they developed the Task Force that accomplished nothing … So I mean the government has shown absolute lack of leadership, in the AIDS epidemic in this province.

During the needs assessment I had the opportunity to interview Eric Smith about the AIDS Task force set up in 1988. He responded:

> The province set up the AIDS task force and I became sort of the token [person living with HIV], you know…. There was about 21 members on it. I was the only one that was infected. There were two other people on it who were gay, but were not publically gay – so I was the token "fairy" as well…. the Task Force has public meetings around the province and public hearings in Halifax. I think I lasted two days … and as the second days was winding up, someone got up and said 'you know I have sat here for six hours … over the last few days, and we have heard all these people talk about what should have been done … we haven't heard anyone talk about what it is like to live with it [HIV] … he said, "my name is [states his own name] and I have AIDS" and he went to say what his life was like.

Most of the activists who were interviewed during the assessment agreed that the failure of the Task Force to meaningfully engage HIV positive gay men crystalized a movement led by people living with HIV. As one of only a small handful of what were termed "PHA-driven organizations" to form in Canada at the time, the Nova Scotia Person with AIDS coalition (NSPWA) was officially registered in 1988 and took as its mandate issues of social support and advocacy, as human rights violations continued to occur. This "safe haven," as some activists referred to it, provided

---

[3] Human T-cell lymphotropic virus/lymphadenopathy (HTLV-LAV) was the first name given to HIV. The virus was isolated by Dr. Robert Gallo of the National Cancer Institute (Glanz 2013).

the environment for members to cultivate their own forms or resistance and launch sometimes subversive social justice projects:

> Well I remember when Dennis was in the hospital, we use to see him and we used to do 24 hour care in the hospital. At one time, there was no home care [services for people dying of AIDS], there was nothing like that and there was very little knowledge, and he was being cared for at home. Finally we decided we couldn't do it, that we didn't have the resources and we didn't have the knowledge or the skills and we took him to the hospital and of course *the hospital wouldn't take him*. We [finally] left him in emergency and walked out. We waited upstairs in the hospital and within a very short time he got a private room and we went back in and visited him and brought him his things. [We were] insisting that staff bring meals in and *put them in the room* as opposed to putting them *by* the door; [We were] getting upset with them, causing a scene and they came in dressed in [protective] suits causing a scene and we wouldn't let them in the rooms sometime. We ripped signs off the door that had the quarantine thing on them. We were just generally a pain in the ass for the hospital and were threatened to be barred by security and telling them to go fuck themselves.

Although such forms of rebellion stood as an open challenge to the state-sponsored health system, in the eyes of reigning public health policy such displays of individual responsibility, community action, and the initiative to create supportive community health environments—discourses which traced back to Lalonde (1974) and re-articulated in the Ottawa Charter in 1986—appeared as exemplary in executing the ideals of health promotion, and thus enabled them to eventually secure their legitimacy within the local health system.[4] This also drew communities into a project in which they increasingly governed themselves and other members of the HIV movement (Rose 1999).

By 1989, NSPWA was granted federal funding along with MACAIDS, which then became AIDS Nova Scotia. While activists credited AIDS Nova Scotia as being, locally, the first to conduct focussed work on "men who have sex with men who did not identify as gay", they viewed AIDS Nova Scotia as a more public health-oriented organization that focused their prevention educational efforts on the "general population." Activists I spoke to were generally critical of their messaging which aimed to de-stigmatize AIDS by asserting the universalistic notion of HIV vulnerability: "AIDS affects everyone." By contrast, NSPWA re-claimed AIDS-related stigma by acknowledging the reality that HIV was mostly affecting people from marginalized communities. NSPWA, according to activists I interviewed for the needs assessment, emphasized targeted work with gay men, women, members of the local black community, and emerging rural communities that had also begun mobilizing responses to the epidemic by the late 1980s and early 1990s.[5]

---

[4] The Lalonde health promotion report rather explicitly opposes health service delivery through technocratic interventions.

[5] Following a national AIDS conference in Vancouver, with growing awareness of the unique HIV vulnerability of indigenous people of Canada, initially 15 First Nations communities from Nova Scotia came together in 1991 and eventually those from across the Atlantic provinces of Canada formed the First Nations AIDS Task Force. Although this entity did over time interact and were allies with ACNS, they operated quite autonomously and therefore did not participate in the provincial needs assessment led by ACNS.

NSPWA's "targeted work" was shaped by what activists were learning of the evolving epidemic in Nova Scotia and beyond. A "state of emergency" arose in Canada and the USA when the rate of reported infections increased most rapidly among women as HIV came to be viewed as a "threat" to the "general population" (Schiller 1992, Schiller et al. 1994). By the early 1990s in Nova Scotia, a growing number of women were being diagnosed with HIV (Allen 1994). Between 1992 and 1993, NSPWA initiated the Nova Scotia Women and AIDS Project throughout Nova Scotia, building networks of women living with HIV and AIDS. This project mobilized the first system of support for women living with HIV and AIDS in Nova Scotia. One of the major themes project coordinator Jane Allen described in her work was that of isolation. These women, she maintained in a 1994 interview, lacked the social networks that gay men readily formed, which drew upon pre-existing gay and lesbian rights networks of the 1970s. She insisted that many women living with AIDS, therefore, suffered in silence while lacking the kind of services that could help ease their experience with the terminal illness. As Allen explained, the isolation experienced by women living with HIV stemmed from the pervasive public perception that HIV was a problem affecting "other groups" such as gay men or injection drug users but not a problem for women; unless a women was a "prostitute or a junkie" she was not viewed as being at risk for HIV infection. In many cases, women who received their diagnosis in the early 1990s did so in the latter and even "full blown" stages of the illness because of how physicians who employed the epidemiologic of risk categories. This was yet another "strike" against biomedicine, as Jane Allen from the Women and AIDS Project explains:

> I think that one of the main differences is that HIV was really framed as a man's disease from day one … so first it was the homosexuals … and then they constructed this thing called the 4-h club, which included homosexuals, hookers,[6] Haitians and haemophiliacs; but for some reason, even when they had this definition of high risk groups, women were never considered as part of those even though women can fall into all of those categories except haemophilia, because it is a male genetic disease; but certainly there are female sex partners of haemophiliacs … Women, in terms of services they can get, are about 10 years behind men even today.
>
> If you are a gay man and you test positive it is a lot easier for you to pick up the phone … and you are probably going to have a lot more support like that around you than if you are a woman in Halifax, Dartmouth or Shelbourne because there isn't the common community … There's also not as much research done on women … and doctors just aren't aware. Very often women get tested a lot, lot *later* … So they often have AIDS before they know they are HIV positive. (Oct. 1994)

Nadine, a woman suffering full blown AIDS at the time I met her, responded to Jane's series of statements during the same interview by saying:

> Yes, that was my main beef … if I could have been tested four or five years ago when I started getting the rashes … and just funny things happened like my appendix broke … there was just a lot of things that happened and if I would've gotten tested, I wouldn't be where I am now … I could've taken better care of myself. AIDS has been defined by high risk groups, but it is not who you are but what you do. (Oct. 1994)

[6] More widely this term for HIV risk groups replaced "hookers" with "heroin addicts" (see for example, Treichler 1999: 51).

Physicians' failure to detect a growing population of women at the earlier stages of HIV sparked the mobilization of a woman's project based on a feminist platform, leading women to seize a space within a predominantly white, gay male activist community to ensure proper treatment and care for women. Similarly, the Black community in Halifax developed a project through ACNS to address the needs of their community. Kimberly Bernard (1993) documented how Black Nova Scotians rejected important HIV prevention information due to suspicions of racism. This perception of racism, she said, resulted from the strong connection that the media was drawing at the time between HIV and its rapid spread and supposed origin in Africa. According to Bernard, the racist assumption that Africans or Black people were somehow the source of contagion caused many African Nova Scotians to disregard information pertaining to HIV and AIDS. The following quotation was taken from a report composed by Bernard for the NSPWA coalition:

> Reports of the rapid spread of AIDS in Africa rely heavily on racist assumptions about African culture. The massive publicity the media gives to the African connection with AIDS makes it evident that black people will suffer emotionally from the speculative and racist comments made by the media health services and scientific community (Bernard, 1993).

During my interview with Bernard, she discussed with me why the project was formed:

> There were several different African Nova Scotians who needed services in relation to HIV and AIDS … there was a lack of comfort, a lack of accessibility, a lack of culturally sensitive materials … so this is how the project was created.

Other grassroots community groups mushroomed across rural geographies of Nova Scotia in the late 1980s and early 1990s, inspired and supported by NSPWA's visible mobilizations of dissent and work with the local news media in Halifax. In addition to gay men, this collective brought together women's groups, members of the Red Cross, which formed palliative care teams, lesbian activists, members of the clergy, and public health nurses.

Despite the difference in philosophy, annual reports from NSPWA and AIDS Nova Scotia from the early 1990s indicate that both organizations maintained considerable ties with each other through volunteer and fund raising activities. In 1993, the two organizations merged their volunteers to coordinate home care services together, sharing the proceeds from fund raising events such as the Silent Wall, Bid for Life Auction, and the yearly AIDS walk. But as AIDS became less of a hot political issue, federal spending was reduced and the two organizations were forced to amalgamate, a process that began in 1994 and was completed on July 1995 with the establishment of the AIDS Coalition of Nova Scotia (ACNS). NSPWAC ideologies won out in the struggle over institutional values and ACNS continued the focus on marginalized groups and maintained the engagement of people living with HIV and AIDS by having a minimum of 51 % representation on the board.

The HIV epidemic in Nova Scotia agitated pre-existing social fissures, making them more pronounced. For gay, lesbian, feminist and black social justice activists and their allies, HIV had become a vehicle to articulate local forms of homophobia, gender inequality, and racism. Consequently, the HIV community response in Halifax continued to evolve through a merging of numerous social movements (though certainly not without their own internal conflicts, at times thorny identity politics and power struggles). Over time, the response had transformed from a grassroots reactive group to a more proactive, lobbying organization, one that continued to extend its network of allies to include government officials, politicians, academic researchers and clinical scientists.

1.3 Community-Based Research

In 1998, Health Canada announced the release of a new program under the third phase of the National AIDS strategy called HIV/AIDS Community-based Research (CBR). This program followed on a series of consultations involving the National Health Research Development Program (NHRDP), the provincial and national representatives from the AIDS Division of Health Canada, and academics and community activists across the country. Soon after the consultation process, various definitions of CBR began to circulate throughout community organizational network channels, including those to which I was connected in Halifax. Important sources of definitions for CBR were inspired by the work of social scientists at the University of Toronto and contract researchers at AIDS Vancouver. Both sources advanced flexible notions of CBR. For example, according to sociologists Allman et al. (1997: 21) of the University of Toronto Epidemiological Unit, CBR was defined as "a philosophy for inquiry and not a discreet research framework… Community-based research may incorporate full action, varying degrees of empowerment, or, at the other extreme, nothing more than the permission of an involved community regarding any one particular research initiative." Adult education scholars, Terry Trussler and Rick Marchand (1998), contracted by AIDS Vancouver, outlined the possible forms of CBR (ranging from organization planning, focus groups, program evaluations, needs assessments, ethno-cultural studies), insisting that CBR was not something new; for community-based organizations (CBOS) across Canada were already undertaking various systematic knowledge production processes.

According to Health Canada program discourse, a "democratized" AIDS research project would be realized through the CBR program, one that would improve the capacity of CBOs to engage in "evidence-based" decision making. What was initially enticing to the community activists I spoke with was how the program rather explicitly acknowledged and legitimated the accumulated experience and practical knowledge that came through working directly with members living with and highly affected by HIV. This program suggested the coming of an epistemological rupture regarding whose knowledge and what types of knowledge could count as authoritative. And activists certainly welcomed this possibility. Already, the ideas of the French social theorist, Michel Foucault, and the links he drew between power and knowledge (Foucault 1980) regularly circulated among members of the HIV movement I spoke with, in the more popularized version—"knowledge *is* power." Activists I spoke with often criticized scientific studies that failed to inform the vital program work they were doing. On one occasion, the home-care coordinator for ACNS said to me

> If I hear about one more epidemiological study that tells us about some fucking [statistical] *association* we already know about.... Like, there was this one study that found a relationship between protease inhibitors and bad tastes and smells. I mean, tell us something we don't know. We know that already—how does that study help us? It just confirms ... what we already know, right![7]

The idea of CBR, of taking the reins of knowledge production processes, therefore was a highly appealing way for activists to envision CBOs as securing greater influence in wider policy arenas. To those working at the grassroots CBO level, "CBR" signalled a transfer of power, in the form of decision making, resources, technology and funding, from the government to "the community." As time would tell, however, what followed was anything but a straightforward transfer of power.

Instead the democratizing process set in motion by the CBR program would be better described as the expansion of state power and the diffusion of an epistemological terrain that re-appraised the value of activists, community members, and movement organizers according to their ability to participate in CBR capacity building activities funded by the program. Nevertheless, this credentialization process, as I came to think of it, neither spelt the erasure of activism nor political dissent. Rather, it transformed the ground on which members realized their roles as activists. As the insights and experiences of the community came to be legitimized in the eyes of the state, I also witnessed how the Health Canada's objective of "building CBR capacity within the CBOs" led to fractures and rearrangements in existing alliances as the formation of new strategic partnerships and collaborations with academics and policy makers, fostered by the Health Canada program, began to crystalize. Meanwhile new forms of exclusion were produced by the growing movement towards "mainstreaming" CBOs within the Canadian public health system.

To recreate some of the conditions that set this credentialization process in motion, I find it helpful to refer to the report written by Terry Trussler and Rick Marchand (1998) entitled "Knowledge from Action: community-based research in Canada's HIV strategy," which presented a conceptual framework for how CBOs could build their capacities to conduct CBR. Although based on the stirrings around CBR in Vancouver, this document was an important initial resource to community HIV researchers throughout Canada, even as far away as Nova Scotia where I conducted my ethnographic study; for it spoke to many of the aspirations of leaders of the community AIDS movement at the time the program was announced. For example, in the forward of the document, AIDS Vancouver executive director at the time, Andrew Johnson comments,[8] optimistically, on Health Canada's new commitment to CBR:

[7] The coordinator was referencing the study by Heald et al. (1998) "Taste and smell complaints in HIV-infected patients."

[8] Andrew Johnson was well known in the HIV movement for having composed the homecare manual, *Living with Dying, Dying at Home*, which he wrote for ACT in 1994. This manual served as a key resource for care team networks that emerged across Canada.

> The potential for community-based research to have an effect on the epidemic is enormous…. We also hope to help prepare community AIDS groups for this research opportunity. A responsive research program must be developed to understand the questions communities want to address…. Like many agencies across the country, AIDS Vancouver has a tradition of doing CBR. That research has often gone unnoticed. We have learned, however, to develop a greater capacity to do research so that our programs and services are more responsive to the communities we serve. We have learned not to make assumptions about who needs our services and what they need.

Such statements indeed resonated with CBOs members across Canada as it evoked notions of producing and owning knowledge that was grounded in the lived experiences of people living with HIV and AIDS.

Vancouver was indeed an important site for the emergence and proliferation of CBR ideologies, serving as a beacon that sparked interest across Canada. This interest was reflected in a special 2-day event at XI international Conference on AIDS in Vancouver in 1996, where more than 40 CBR practitioners from across the globe came together to establish a consensus around a CBR strategy for HIV/AIDS. Sharing their experiences, it was clear that many were working in isolation. In this way CBR as a political ideology was highly effective in connecting a global network of social actors with overlapping epistemological concerns related to the nature of knowledge required to improve epidemic prevention.

In 1999, I attended a CBR national workshop hosted by AIDS Vancouver. One of the trainers, sociologist Dan Allman, led the multiple members of CBOs and their allied researchers (like me), through an impressive and in-depth process of defining "what is CBR?". In small groups we all came up with extensive definitions that emphasized "community wisdom"—the knowledge that came from our experiences of directly working with and learning from the struggles of those who were living with HIV. In one of the small discussion groups, a CBO executive director, representing an indigenous First Nations community, turned to the group and rather adamantly said "I am just tired of reading these damn epidemiological studies that tell you about some association or correlation they've discovered that we already know about." The conversation that followed then turned to "sample size" as another member claimed he knew better, through his work, the needs and problems facing people living with HIV compared to health scientists because he was in regular contact with hundreds of people living with HIV: "I have a big enough 'sample size' to know!" Some discussion of this statement ensued. Eventually a consensus was reached: although many of us may have had the ear of the community and an intimate knowledge of daily lived experiences of people living with HIV, we needed to be "more systematic" in how we understand and analysed the needs of "the community." As a social worker doing his PhD with a HIV community-based organization, one participant said "we need to be careful *not* to assume we know all the needs of the community without systematically gathering data and analysing the data." The small group agreed.[9]

---

[9] CATIE began as an initiative of the grassroots group AIDS Action Now, located in Toronto's gay village. It responded to the growing demand for lay-friendly treatment information. In addition to producing and disseminating accessible treatment information, such as those that reached ACNS they also provided a treatment information hotline.

Similar discussions appeared in the Health Canada's consultations around CBR with CBOs in the lead up to the third iteration of the National AIDS strategy (Trussler and Marchand 1998: 2). Trussler and Marchand (1998), in support of the government initiative, outlined a series of justifications for enhancing CBR capacity building in Canadian CBOs, based on the discussions that grew out of the nation-wide consultation process. I present here a series of abbreviated excerpts and some critical commentary to highlight the key logics that helped to usher CBR into the domain of community politics and action.

(i) "Community experience & information: Valuable information on local epidemiological dynamics exists in the experience and records of community agencies.... Building the research capacities of community AIDS groups would enable them to provide the data on critical trends to health authorities. If heeded, this evidence could ensure a more timely and effective response to early warning signs."

Here the idea is that there are prized pockets of knowledge that exist outside the view of public health; such grounded knowledge could more effectively tip off health authorities in the case of emerging epidemics. Importantly, the implicit suggestion here is that CBOs can play a more central role in epidemiological tracking and surveillance, given their empirical "location." The phrase "more timely" suggests that community knowledge can also help in creating more efficient modes of HIV surveillance, where on-the-ground detection can more speedily transport local knowledge to the concentrated centres of public health authority.

(ii) "Mobilizing HIV Health Promotion: Community organizations need good information about the social environment to interest, motivate and mobilize their populations for HIV health promotion.... Enhanced research activities would not only help provide needed evidence for confident decision making, but also important tools and skills for active meaningful and convincing participation in community health efforts."

This excerpt suggests that through CBR activities contextual knowledge could be generated to aid in CBO health promotional activities. Producing such knowledge is possible for CBOs, of course, because of their being embedded in the lived realities of highly affected communities. Thus, CBR knowledge production regimes are imagined here as capitalizing on the social affinities, solidarities and relations of trust, forged out of forms of activism that once stood in radical opposition to governmental and biomedical institutions—for the (normative) public health prescription of health promotion.

(iii) "Community practise: building the capacity for research builds the general capacities of HIV/AIDS agencies."

The suggestion here is that learning, functioning (and perhaps even becoming) more like researchers, would foster more effective ways to lead the community-level response. This characterization reiterates the role of CBOs in the response as (needing to be) centred around systematized knowledge production processes, as though the effectiveness of CBOs lies in their ability to produce and utilize formalized knowledge.

(iv) "Research participation: [CBR] would allow better information flow between researchers and communities. Academic researchers will recognize new opportunities to tap into community knowledge available from skilled community-based researchers and frontline workers. A national network of qualified community-based research personnel would create an effective liason between vulnerable communities and clinical, epidemiological and social scientists."

CBR is portrayed as establishing an information highway that provides direct access to hidden knowledge imagined to reside at "the grassroots."

Although this document maintains the imaginary of social and political "margins" and "centres," I would insist, the CBR program signified the expansion of the state's agency within a new (and more intimate) territory that further entangled diverse grouping of activists, researchers, health officials that reference "evidence production" itself as a justification for its power. Although the Marchand and Trussler report valorizes "evidence-based decision making"—a policy discourse that was firmly tied to notions of accountability between Health Canada as a funder and CBO funding recipients—the question of what counted as "evidence" was left relatively open to the interpretation of multiple academic disciplines. In fact, Marchand and Trussler supported the importance of qualitative studies, which CBOs leader called for during the consultation "to unpack the demographic and epidemiological data that are circulated to communities" (10). Critically, they acknowledge that "qualitative research paradigms continue to meet with confusion and scepticism. Few people are able to move comfortably between qualitative and quantitative methods." Acknowledging that CBOs throughout Canada had conducted their share of "smaller scale" studies, Trussler and Marchard characterized these collective CBO activities as "unguided", "uncoordinated" and having "little monitoring of nation-wide knowledge development at the community level." Thus, they imagine CBR as needing to become a more streamlined, efficient, and nationally coordinated machine.

Next I present three ethnographic sketches of knowledge production processes that were inspired and animated by the promotion of CBR. From the perspective of my role as the provincial needs assessment coordinator I illustrate how the quest for hidden knowledge at the grassroots eventually guided communities of people injecting drugs into a series of CBR capacity building meetings that inadvertently tore apart social solidarities at the same time as new strategic alliances were sutured together in the name of CBR.

1.3.1 "Hidden" Knowledges

When I came to coordinate the NS province-wide needs assessment for ACNS in 1998, part of my responsibility was to interview members working in CBOs in the small urban settings of Sydney and North Sydney, Cape Breton. In my home town of Sydney, a needle exchange office had recently been built next to the AIDS coalition to accommodate an HIV-hepatitis C outbreak (Lior et al. 1998), which mostly affected poor and working class heterosexual men and women, some of whom sold sex. The island of Cape Breton had one of the highest unemployment rates in the country. Naturally deep harbours coupled with the receding presence of the national police, the Royal Canadian Mounted Police, made Sydney and North Sydney harbours an ideal entry point for importing illicit drugs into Canada. Injection drug use and the concomitant HIV-HCV (hepatitis C virus) epidemics were linked together through the thriving drug trade, as local needle exchange staff and people using injection drugs explained to me.

During my first visit to the needle exchange I met with the CBO executive director, who self-identified as a gay man. He then introduced me to Barbara, an outreach worker in her mid-30s, who greeted me by saying, "I hear you are an anthropologist. I'm a Marxist feminist." With enthusiasm, she expressed her desire to take me into the field to meet with members of the injection drug using community so that I might better understand the context in which people were using drugs. While smiling, she said "We really need to do an ethnographic study here because there is so much knowledge that no one knows about, except for us!"

Barbara then explained how she was able to gain rapport and entree into the daily lives of the people to whom she gave clean needles, "Well Robert, I sometime will take a drag [a puff of marijuana] and they see that and they know that I can be trusted, that I am not judging them— but don't tell Health Canada!" she said while laughing. As we drove to one member's house, she explained that there had been some murders and a number of other crimes that could be traced back to people who accessed the needle exchange services "But you know, we have a good relationship with the police. They'll see our [bright yellow] sharp containers at members' homes and they won't get arrested cause they know [these people injecting drugs] are being responsible."

During my first interview with Barbara she explained how her "community approach" differed from a "public health approach":

> We are a community organization that is serving people in a way that does not judge people. We don't come at them with the wagging finger telling them "you shouldn't be, you shouldn't be" and we take people exactly where they are. I generally spend 45 minutes with each person … its educating and just chatting and support. Some of the people there are injection drug users; they are at high risk for infection … so what I talk to them about is continuing the harm reduction perspective; try to help them with a plan. But it is difficult to urge people to get tested when you tell them that they will also be recorded by the department of health.

Continuing to explain the motivations underlying her commitment to this work, Barbara said:

> When I see people who are HIV+ and they are coming through the door for clean needles … that's when I know they have a good supply, and they are travelling in different circles. That's what keeps you going. For example 12,000 needles came in the other day from this site and there is a couple of people who are HIV positive in that community and so you know that these needles are not going to be dispersed and these needles are going to be off the street and they have more supplies … you know that it is working.

Barbara explained that there were particular problems that had emerged out of locating the needle exchange next to an AIDS coalition run by gay and lesbian people.

> Sometimes different people over the phone who use injection drugs told me they would never come into the needle exchange and they say … "Oh they're all gay" and "I don't want to be labelled"…. But you see many of these people who do use injection drugs have been sexually abused as children and anybody who is gay is a child molester in their heads … they consider homosexuals as a potential threat.

As I was to learn, this community of people using drugs commonly associated "homosexuality" with sex between inmates. This knowledge formed a silent but shared reality among those who had been incarcerated. Barbara pointed out an interesting irony to me one day when we were visiting a few men who had found themselves imprisoned in a local correction facility. She pointed to the wall that said "sex between inmates is prohibited" and below it was another make-shift sign that said "condoms are available at the nurses' station." This irony not only pointed to the reality that inmates had sex with each other; it was also indicative of the prohibitive regime around which same-sex sexual relations were cast, a regime that markedly contrasted with the queer discourse of freedom that conditioned the visibility of sexualities reflected in the adjacent AIDS coalition.

Irony and "the unexpected" were a regular part of doing outreach work among people injecting drugs, Barbara explained. This became clear when she took me on a visit to meet with a young mid 20 year old woman, Tanya, who had recently lost her infant to child social services. We arrived at a small house with an annoyed looking older man waiting at the door in the upstairs unit. Barb explained that that he was the landlord—"a slum-lord"—she called him, who had stopped paying for the hot water and heat on Tanya's unit because he knew she was using drugs and selling sex in the downstairs unit. The man also forced Tanya to provide him with "sexual favours," Barb said.

That day, the landlord knew that Barb was coming to help Tanya move out of the very dark and cold basement apartment and he scowled at us from his inside his door. Indeed this was the cause that Barb, the self-declared Marxist feminist was waiting for. After helping Tanya pack her belongings in the car, we all headed to Tanya's new home, which the AIDS coalition and needle exchange had arranged through their partnership with local social services agencies. The new place was clean and brightly lit. A box with a disassembled crib lay against the wall. Barb called on one of the volunteers, Tim, to meet us at Tanya's home. Tim introduced himself to me as a "recovering addict." As an experienced carpenter, he quickly and nimbly set up the crib. Barb and I left that Friday feeling rather satisfied with a job well done. The following Monday when I followed up on how Tanya was doing, Barb shook her head at me, with a rather perplexed expression while telling me that Tanya and Tim "went on a drug run all weekend and spent all the rent money. Now she's been evicted from the new place because of all the partying and noise." Barb continued, "Sometimes, I have no idea why I am doing this work!"

But Barb's hesitancy and uncertainty only wavered momentarily. By readily building rapport with the community of people injecting drugs she was able to advocate for their more direct involvement in service delivery. She often referred to members who volunteered at the needle exchange as "natural helpers" given their direct connection to and participation in drug using networks.[10] She mentioned during an interview that "they are the ones who truly know the needs of the community. *They have the real knowledge*, right? So we need to learn from *them,* how to serve the community."

Soon a recovering addict named Dan was hired on a part-time, voluntary basis at the needle exchange. He was a very friendly and likeable guy who, because of his new volunteer position, decided to start a Bachelor of Arts in community development at the local university. During an interview with Dan he discussed his work with the needle exchange:

> I run into a few people I know here [at the needle exchange]. I've been in the prison system so my experience is valuable to the clients … as an addict, I know that I can't change a person … I can't preach to someone why it is bad for them to do something. But if you are going to do something' let's keep it safe as possible … so you don't get sick or don't pass it to someone else. So we keep it on that level and if they want to go on a different level and ask me about recovery and how I'm doing it, then of course I'll go there with them … because I have experience.

At the same time, Dan mentioned how his work as a "natural helper" also posed a challenge for his addiction recovery process:

> It contradicts a lot of the recovery issues because I have to be one of the guys again and you get back into using the lingo … so I guess it keeps you on your toes with your recovery … you don't want to go back to that … I have to keep in touch with my support network. I try to give the clients myself and can provide insights if they want them from my own experience, into recovery.

In her ongoing efforts to recruit "natural helpers" to help deliver programs and services at the needle exchange, Barb worked hard to build trust with one person in particular—Mary, who identified as a lesbian, and as a former sex worker. At the time, she was running a brothel and escort agency next to a large Catholic church. Mary was particularly prized in the eyes of Barb because she has been part of the drug and sex worker networks for many years and she was viewed as possessing specialized knowledge that no one else did. I was invited to interview Mary in her

---

[10] The natural helper model and program are further described in the following short document: http://www.med.mun.ca/getdoc/f05fb23e-2500-46bd-8cb9-2bf737ae7033/NaturalHelperManual.aspx

home surrounded by abundant couches, with young women coming and going, treating the madam with a mixture of fear and reverence as though she were their mother and abuser. Barb was thrilled that the interview we conducted captured very detailed knowledge about local drug using networks and risk. During the interview Mary explained to us:

> The hard core group knows who is positive, but they do not seemed that concerned … they figure it's too late, they've been [sharing needles] together for year; so if one's got it I've got it, so who care anyways. Most of them assume they've got it, even if there is denial; it's a sort of given. You Know if "so and so's" got it and I've been banging with him for several years, so I must have it. The core group I see is kind of hopeless…. They figure that they are drug addicts and they are going to stay drug addicts … AIDS is just a risk that goes along with using … the majority are not going to get tested even though their boyfriend or girlfriend test positive.
>
> The border group, the recreational or occasional users are a lot more concerned. They have jobs, they have families, they have children … they have things to loose … but when they get high it goes out the window; they are more careful than core users. People come here in the middle of the night for condoms or clean needles … there's no questions asked. People are taking good advantage of the needle exchange, but when it's the middle of the night and they've run out…. It's back to using old needles.

It was this kind of "hidden knowledge" that Mary shared that led her to become an important volunteer for the organization. In a closed meeting with the AIDS coalition and needle exchange staff, Mary and a few other people who injected drugs were granted centre stage to instruct staff and the board members, based on their experiences, and advise on the ways to properly "reach" these communities. Because of the specialized knowledge they demonstrated during the needs assessment, such "natural helpers" came to play a central role in the community-based research capacity building initiative, which was beginning to unfold.

1.4 Shifting Networks

Health Canada eventually granted CBR funds to ACNs through a capacity building call announced in 1998. ACNS generously created the position of research director for me, with the main responsibility of coordinating CBR capacity building activities in Nova and across the Atlantic provinces, a process which eventually took the form of a series of community research training sessions. For the Atlantic Canada training sessions, academic researchers provided a series of training workshops on how to construct a research question, the difference between qualitative and quantitative research, mixed methodologies, and so on. Three of the CBO directors were themselves in the process of completing PhD programs, and were adamant in saying to the workshop facilitator I had hired for the workshops "We don't want a lot of process!" Thumbing their noses at the adult educational learning approach that the facilitator was adhering to, they said, instead, "We want content!" Tension emerged among the CBR training participants over this issue. The director for an HIV/AIDS indigenous people's organization very diplomatically put it "I don't mind all the process because I am not a researcher and I need to be led through this, as it is new for me, and some of the others".

This tension never resolved itself but what became clear was the jockeying for power, and the uneven sense of comfort that the Atlantic workshop participants held in relation to the CBR capacity building project. A bifurcation between two "tiers" of participants became apparent through this process. Divisions also formed along epistemological lines. At one point in a conversation about "community wisdom", a highly regarded outreach worker at ACNS was asked about his "strategies" for reaching men in cruising spots, under the assumption that his approaches could be applied to research recruitment. Tom's response was telling: "Um … Ah… [he hesitates for some time]. I don't know if I really have any "strategy"; I mean these are the men that I fuck; they are my peers, you know, so I give them information. But it is not formal."

Similarly, when I was asked to temporarily fill in for Tom for the MSM (men who have sex with men) Outreach Project in 1998 as the acting training coordinator, I used to go to clubs and other places where my peers congregated. Here the kind of knowledge and approach I took, while intent on informing and connecting men to STI services at the anonymous clinic housed at ACNS, was also highly "informal" in the sense that it was inseparable from the social context, making it impossible to articulate a "method" or "strategy" apart from the myriad subtleties of social engagement. I would have stumbled too, like Innis, if asked to detail how I connected these men. This kind of informal practical "know how" seemed quite different from the formal research methodologies being introduced through the CBR capacity building workshops. The workshops advanced "methods" for recruiting participants as if these techniques were ontologically independent from social contexts. Nevertheless, despite Innis' moment of hesitation and uncertainty, the CBR training carried on as though informal ways of knowing and doing could be readily formalized and standardized to serve the interests of public health research.

In reflecting on this process of knowledge formalization, I have come to think about the CBR capacity building workshops as a process of epistemological transfiguration—that is, as a process that mines and refines informal knowledges and practises, purifying them to serve the "elevated" and standardized order of Health Science. The religious connotation here is deliberate as I want to highlight the intensely moral compulsion I witnessed surrounding this process, which was evident in the considerable devotion displayed to community-based research on the part of CBOs leaders and staff across Canada at that moment in time.

With respect to the internal provincial CBR capacity building meetings that I coordinated under the supervision of CBO directors in Nova Scotia, the fracturing of affective networks and solidarities became even more pronounced, as the following fieldnote excerpt illustrates:

> *After lunchtime on the third day of the second round of CBR capacity building training, held in Halifax, I saw Dan sitting by himself looking quite upset, on the verge of tears. Knowing Dan quite well, I approached him and asked what was upsetting him. He burst into tears (something I never seen him do in my two years of knowing him, even under the most dis-*

turbing of conditions that periodically arose at the needle exchange) and exclaimed "my marriage is ruined because of that fucking Mary!"

Dan recounted his life story to me during the conversation, describing himself as a recovered cocaine addict. He said he had finally gotten his life together after "hitting rock bottom", which almost cost him his life. In his late 30s, he decided to pursue a university education and was in his second year of completing his community development services. Several researchers, coalition board members involved in the CBR capacity building process were keen to recruit Dan for several reasons: for one, he was no longer using; he was highly intelligent, friendly and easy to work with; and he remained well-connected to the community of people injecting drugs through his part-time work at the needle exchange in Cape Breton. In sum, he appeared as the ideal kind of community worker for the injection drug community in the era of CBR.

Mary, on the other hand, was still "using', was actively involved in sex work as a madam and frequently showed up intoxicated for meetings. Nevertheless Coalition staff and board members were always impressed with Mary because of her compelling stories that detailed recitations of insider knowledge. Like Dan she was recognized within community activist networks as highly insightful and a leader. During the capacity building project it became apparent that those like Dan who were more "recovered" would gain some type of paid work out of the process and play a leading role in future CBR activities. Those like Mary, on the other hand were expected to participate in CBR projects in a more voluntary role. According to Dan, Mary was jealous of him because he was receiving so much praise for "cleaning up his life" and going back to university. He insisted that Mary thought he "no longer represented the community" because he had gone "straight" [stopped using drugs].

On this day just before lunch, Mary had gone out and returned with another woman who was not part of the workshop series. This woman knew Dan quite well although he had not seen her for years since he was using. Dan explained that the woman proceeded to tell his wife how she and Dan were connected in the past. The woman told Dan's wife that he was formerly a "male prostitute" who worked for her escort agency. Dan's wife was so upset, he told me, that she left Halifax and returned to Cape Breton without him. As Dan continued the story, he explained that Mary was the reason he "hit bottom". While he worked at her escort agency, he and Mary had fought over money. According to Dan, Mary used a baseball bat to bludgeon him on the head repeatedly until, as he described it, she had "blackened my skull", landing him in the hospital. This was the event, Dan explained, that forced him turn his life around. But now, with his wife so angry, he said he felt like he was 'right back there again,' he said. Thus he felt he was no longer 'recovered.' He couldn't imagine his wife would stay with him after finding out what had happened.

During the provincial CBR capacity building training session, tensions between workshop participants began to grow in relation to how the workshop activities were organized with respect to time. A number of the participants who injected drugs, and who were at various stages of recovery, exited the room every 20 min or so to get a "fix." A few of the more middle class gay participants became outraged at these individuals, and some went as far as accusing them of being "uncommitted activists." Thus the temporal aspects of the workshops unintentionally created inclusions and exclusion groups based on the degree which people struggled with their dependency and addictions. In other words, "ideal participation"—in the manner it was constructed in and through CBR capacity building—began to tear apart the very bonds of solidarity that held together this community.

***

In their discussion of scientific citizenship, Adrian Guta and colleagues (2014: 258) describe how Canada's CBR initiative served to discipline community participation while extending "the state's ability to strategically manage policy decisions." My depictions of the CBR capacity building process contribute to this picture of subjectification by showing how communities become drawn into the governmental project of managing the health of "vulnerable groups" through the production of the knowledge that counted in HIV health policy domains. The effectiveness of this program to some extent lays in its ability to affect and embroil a range of social actors—from CBO executive directors working on PhD projects, to outreach workers like Barbara and natural helpers, like Dan and Mary—in the goals of the program. Their passionate engagements feeds into a mode of evidentiary sovereignty that allows for recognition of an array of evidence, which includes an appreciation for qualitative information and the kinds of "insider" narratives that frontline members of the HIV movement exchange with each other. Thus the ability of this program to extend Health Canada's authority into the intimate social textures of the HIV movement took place through a vehicle of 'democratic' participation, rather than vertical imposition from Health Canada.

However, I would insist that this movement of power cannot be entirely understood as a progressive transition from a radical form of activism to one that is rendered docile, normalized, and coopted by the Health Canada program, as such a storyline inevitably lapses into an uncritical nostalgia. Instead, this mode of sovereignty operated by redefining the very boundaries of community participation in the HIV movement, as some activists, members, and community health workers came to be viewed as more legitimately suited to participate in the CBR program compared to others. In other words, this story must also be understood as a tale of expulsion;[11] those unable to meet the new demands of the evidentiary sovereign become expelled from the territory of the HIV response.

Attention to the history of the shifting affective connections of the HIV movement in Nova Scotia reveals how transformations in the era of CBR arrives by excluding perspectives and lived realities of importance for understanding the struggles with the HIV epidemic. Such abjection was a crucial part of how some members were able to more forcefully re-position themselves in policy arenas, re-asserting their identities as activists in the era of neoliberal policy reforms that emphasized population health perspectives and evidence-based decision making over community health promotion.

[11] My thinking here owes much to Kristeva's notion of abjection and her discussion in *Powers of Horror* (1980) of how disavowal, rejection, and expulsion are inherent to the process of becoming a subject (Kristeva 1980).

References

Allen, J. (1994). *Women and HIV/AIDS in Nova Scotia: Needs assessment report. Nova Scotia women and AIDS project.* Halifax: The AIDS Coalition of Nova Scotia.

Allman, D., Myers, T., & Cockerill, R. (1997). *Concepts, definitions and models for community-based HIV prevention research in Canada, and, a planning guide for the development of community-based prevention research.* Toronto: HIV Social, Behavioural and Epidemiological Studies Unit, Faculty of Medicine, University of Toronto.

Bernard, K. (1993, August 30). *Community AIDS Education for the African Nova Scotian Community: Needs assessment report.* Halifax: Nova Scotia Persons with AIDS Coalition Black Outreach Project.

Foucault, M. (1980). *Power/knowledge: Selected interviews and other writings, 1972–1977.* New York: Pantheon.

Glanz, V. (2013). *History of AIDS.* Delaware: Grand Union University.

Guta, A., Strike, C., Flicker, S., Murray, S. J., Upshur, R., & Myers, T. (2014). Governing through community-based research: lessons from the Canadian HIV research sector. *Social Science & Medicine, 123*, 250–261.

Heald, A. E., Pieper, C. F., & Schiffman, S. S. (1998). Taste and smell complaints in HIV-infected patients. *AIDS, 12*(13), 1667–1674.

Jones, D., & Sheppard, N. C. (1989). AIDS and Disability Employment Discrimination in and beyond the classroom. *Dalhousie* Law Journal, *12*, 103.

Kristeva, J. (1980). *Powers of Horror: An Essay on Abjection.* (Leon S. Roudiez, Trans.). New York: Columbia University Press, (1982). Print. Trans. of *Pouvoirs de l'horreur.* Paris: Editions du Seui.

Lalonde, M. (1974). *A new perspective on the health of Canadians.* Ottawa: Information Canada. http://www.phac-aspc.gc.ca/ph-sp/pdf/perspect-eng.pdf.

Lior, L., Stratton, E., & Archibald, C. P., et al. (1998). *Eastern Region Project: Seroprevalence of HIV, HBV, and HCV viruses and high risk behaviours among IDU and sexual partners of IDU.* Slide presentation, Health Canada.

Murray, S. J. (2008). Thanatopolitics: Reading in Agamben a rejoinder to biopolitical life. *Communication and Critical/Cultural Studies, 5*(2), 203–207.

Numer, M. (2014). *Gay men's sexual subjectivities in the age of HIV/AIDS: A poststructural discourse analysis of activists' experiences in Nova Scotia.* Unpublished Ph.D. Thesis. Halifax: Dalhousie University.

Rose, N. (1999). *Powers of freedom: Reframing political thought.* Cambridge: Cambridge University Press.

Schiller, N. G. (1992). What's wrong with this picture? The hegemonic construction of culture in AIDS research in the United States. *Medical Anthropology Quarterly, 6*(3), 237–254.

Schiller, N. G., Crystal, S., & Lewellen, D. (1994). Risky business: The cultural construction of AIDS risk groups. *Social Science & Medicine, 38*(10), 1337–1346.

Stoller, N. E. (1998). *Lessons from the damned: Queers, whores, and junkies respond to AIDS.* New York: Psychology Press.

Treichler, P. A. (1999). *How to have theory in an epidemic: Cultural chronicles of AIDS.* Durham: Duke University Press.

Trussler, T., & Marchand, R. (1998). *Knowledge from action: Community-based research in Canada's HIV strategy.* Vancouver: AIDS Vancouver.

World Health Organization (WHO). (1986). *Ottawa charter for health promotion.* Geneva: WHO.

Chapter 2
Treatment Rebellions

Abstract Transformations in HIV activism in Nova Scotia transpired around the release of a new class of anti-retroviral therapies in late 1995. Decreases in mortality and the extension of life did not spell the death of social dissent, but transformed it into bodily rebellions as members of the local HIV movement confronted onerous treatment regimens, with a multitude of pills, and inconsistent effectiveness from the earliest versions of combination therapy. As this chapter illustrate, these conflicts with biomedicine were less visible to the public than previous protests, playing out at the level of body, as activists spent more and more time negotiating the quality of their lives and futures with medical professionals. From 1995 until 1998, exchanges between HIV positive activists shifted existential questions pivoting around concerns of "when will I die?" to "how do I live well?" Amid these emergent struggles, experimental drugs opened up a new frontier for activism as a clinical trials community began to form and people living with HIV and AIDS came to sit on regulatory boards to influence the protocols surrounding the circulation and "compassionate release" of new and experimental medicines.

Keywords Clinical trials • Antiretrovirals • Canada • 1990s • Treatment activism • History of HIV treatment

> Small preliminary studies that will be reported this week at a national medical meeting show that a new class of drugs is highly effective in knocking out the virus that causes AIDS and allowing the immune system to recover….
>
> The new results are from studies with protease inhibitors, drugs that block a key viral enzyme. The drugs currently on the market block a different enzyme, reverse transcriptase, and these drugs are generally acknowledged to be weak, at best, in staunching the progress of infection with H.I.V., the virus that causes AIDS. But the protease inhibitors appear different. Dr. George Shaw of the University of Alabama at Birmingham said the new results were "groundbreaking."
>
> –Gina Kolata, *New York Times*, 1995,
>
> [http://www.nytimes.com/1995/01/29/us/researchers-find-early-battlers-of-hiv.html]

R. Lorway, *AIDS Activism, Science and Community Across Three Continents*, Social Aspects of HIV 1, DOI 10.1007/978-3-319-42199-5_2

> Indeed, in early trials in AIDS patients, orally administered ABT-538 [Ritonavir] has produced profound declines in plasma viral RNA with concomitant increases in CD4 cells. The continued investigation of ABT-538 for treatment of HIV infection is therefore strongly warranted.
>
> —Kempf et al. 1995

Further transformations in HIV activism in Nova Scotia transpired with the release of a new class of anti-retroviral (ARV) therapies in late 1995. Decreases in mortality and the extension of life did not spell the death of social dissent, but transformed it into bodily rebellions as members of ACNS confronted onerous treatment regimens, with a multitude of pills, and inconsistent effectiveness from the earliest versions of combination therapy, between 1995 and 1998. These emergent struggles with biomedicine were less visible to the public than previous protests, playing out at the level of body, as activists spent more and more time negotiating the quality of their lives and futures with medical professionals. The community of people living with HIV I came to know in Halifax came to reimagine activism as their lives became increasingly entangled in the experimental futures of clinical trials.

In *Impure Science* (1996: 281), sociologist Stephen Epstein describes the intense interest that US AIDS activists paid to the scientific reports of new treatment findings in the early 1990s. I similarly observed this intense interest among many of the activists of ACNS living with HIV during my volunteer work there. Between 1995 and 1997, I helped to update and organize the treatment and clinical trial results briefs that the Canadian AIDS Treatment Information Exchange, a community-based organization, made available to AIDS service organizations across Canada. Members of ACNS not only kept close track of the results of new ARVs that were in various stages of testing, but also closely followed the results of experimental treatments for opportunistic infections, as well as the findings from vitamin and herbal clinical trials.

The discovery of a new class of highly active anti-retrovirals (HAART) in 1995 sent the largest surge of enthusiasm across the networks of AIDS activists in Halifax. I remember clearly the expression on Wilson Hodder's face in late August 1995, when he eagerly showed me the faxed copy of a research paper he had obtained on ABT-538 (also known as ritonavir) authored by the scientist Kempf and colleagues (1995) (excerpted above). Wilson was beaming as he took me through the highlights of the findings. He began speaking about the impressively "high absorption rate" of the drugs when taken orally and the success not only "in vitro" and in animals studies but also in human participants. "With most of the drugs now they don't absorb in the body well and get metabolized by the liver too quickly. This [ritonavir] is going to change everything!" he declared. And in the coming years, much did change for the members of ACNS who were living with HIV and AIDS.

The subsequent release of this new class of anti-retroviral medications represented a major turning point not only in HIV treatment science but also in AIDS activism. This chapter continues the story of how the vitality of AIDS activism and the culture of dissent co-evolved with treatment advancements during this period. As discussed in the previous chapter, increasing entanglements in the state bureaucratic apparatus had already begun reshaping the social arrangement of the community-level response. At the same time, the release of new and experimental drugs began to reroute the force of protestation toward the body, in a manner that individualized HIV positive members' experiences, at the same time as it renewed collective concerns. The release of new and experimental drugs created a diversity of experiences and struggles with demanding regimens, inconsistent effectiveness and side-effects, and emerging insurance problems. From 1995 until 1998, I witnessed how the exchanges between HIV positive members of ACNS shifted existential questions pivoting around concerns of "when will I die?" to "how do I live *well*?" Amid these emergent struggles, experimental drugs also opened up a new frontier for activism as a clinical trials community began to form and people living with HIV and AIDS came to sit on regulatory boards to influence the protocols surrounding the circulation and "compassionate release" of new and experimental medicines.

2.1 Treatment Conflicts

According to "the book" close to the front desk at ACNS, which listed the dates when members died, the mortality rate of HIV markedly declined between 1996 and 1998. When visitors from the public, media or government entered the offices of ACNS, the rather perky office administrator, sometimes tossing his long blond ringlets about, would tell them that "Everyone is doing well around here!" And dramatic success stories certainly circulated throughout the membership, such as in the two narratives that follow.

Sam, who was a visual artist and school teacher, describes the significant impact of the protease inhibitors:

> I didn't get tested until I came down with pneumonia, January 93 … so I found out I had AIDS before I found out I was HIV positive… it was PCP [Pneumocystis pneumonia] … they did a T-cell count … it came back at 65 which is extremely low which means that I was positive for a long, long time. I was lucky to survive this pneumonia. In talking with the doctors [I asked] "How long?" They said, "Where you are with your T-cells and your health … you will have six months."
>
> I was on AZT for a while. I think the next one was 3TC … it was just monotherapy [single drug therapy] at that time. AZT didn't agree with me at all. I finally stopped taking AZT after a year. Starting at 65 [T-cells], I went up to 150, and then down to 100 and then it just never went above 100 again. It kept going down again lower and lower … and then it bottomed out at 7 [T-cells].
>
> Protease inhibitors changed my life! I'll tell you why, because my viral load was a so high, like 584,000 [particles per ml]. It was so high that I felt like I was fighting something every day of my life … it was so debilitating. I slept too much … I couldn't move … there was always nausea there … I was just really sick. In the middle of 96 … I started taking the first cocktail which was ritonavir … the protease inhibitor I started with. It was very difficult to take … it was really wretched stuff, but I was really determined to make it work. So, I did it and I felt miserable and about one and one half months into it … I just woke up one morning and I just felt like a million bucks. I wasn't fighting something anymore. I felt like it was being eradicated. I was so excited about that … I thought, "well, maybe my eyes will be able to come back [Sam had CMV retinitis][1] …. Now everything is going to be fixed!" It

[1] Cytomegalovirus is a form of the herpes virus that can cause retinitis, a degenerative eye disease that can lead to cause visual impairment.

was only then that I could entertain the idea of *doing* something … I could commit myself to doing something. So that's when I started to volunteer and work here at ACNS.

Nadine, who I first met shortly after she had been diagnosed with what doctors referred to as "full blown AIDS," similarly spoke of the life-altering effects of protease inhibitors:

When I was first diagnosed … I was diagnosed at 80 [T-cells]. At one point I was hospitalized for a month. I tried AZT … it didn't work. Over a five year period I've tried everything … nothing worked. I couldn't keep it down [because of] the side effects. And then the protease inhibitors came out. The first one I tried was Crixivan … I had a major reaction … I went off that … I tried a bit of everything and nothing was working … so my doctor suggested I just go to palliative care.... I was under palliative for a while. So then I started to feel a bit better, but I said "No!" I was not satisfied that someone was telling me there was nothing left to try.... so I went back and I changed my doctor.... He had a few more combinations. They weren't working at first but then I started gaining weight and I was feeling better. So now I'm on saquinavir, ritonavir and d4T [combination therapy].... I'm doing great now … I'm up to 500 and my viral load is undetectable. Five years ago I feared I was dying … now it's like, Oh my god can they cut off my Canada pension [said jokingly]? … then I will die [laughing] (Sept. 1998)

As both Sam and Nadine's narratives show, "treatment success" was not without its complications, particularly at a time when many of the newly released drugs were still under refinement with respect to dosage and combination. During this experimental period, those taking new mediations often encountered severe and multiple side-effects—realities which greatly affected their quality of life.

At the time I conducted fieldwork, the successes that members did report were often short lived. For instance, a few months later, Sam reported his treatment failure:

Presently I'm taking d4T and ddI … it's probably actually going to be changed this week because my T-cells are going down and my viral load is increasing … it doesn't seem like it is working. (Sept- 1998)

My time spent talking with members and staff of ACNS led me to the realization that the notion of a "Lazarus effect"—a dramatic return to life from the brink of death—did not entirely characterize people who were sick with AIDS taking protease inhibitor combinations. The treatment narratives of many of these people did not express straightforward "success stories." Larry, for instance, described his experience with the new combinations therapies around the same time period:

There was a lot of hope about these medications [protease inhibitors]…I think for some people, for a good amount of people it saved their lives.... For me, they've … they've done what they are supposed to do … keep me at base.... But my life hasn't gotten any better in terms of my physical health.... I'm no better than I was four years ago.…

I've seen people that were on their deathbed and come out of it and that's excellent and great and I think that research is moving forward and I hope … I don't have any hope for a cure. I think they will probably come up with a vaccine for people that aren't infected and then keep us going and going with new treatments.

The first protease inhibitor I went on was ritonavir … because, after the opportunistic infection [herpes simplex down the oesophagus and stomach], my T-cell count was so low and my viral load so high. So ritonavir, as was my understanding from reading … it was the first resort pill. It was the most powerful thing they gave me. And the side effects were out of this world … the worst pill I'd ever taken; on the other hand, it brought my T-cell count up and my viral load went undetectable, but I had to stop it eventually because of the side effects.

I'm on d4T and saquinavir right now. That's done absolutely nothing for me! I'm where I'm at a year ago when I started. Probably one of the reasons is that you're supposed to take grapefruit juice with it.... There is an enzyme in grapefruit juice, it helps digest, assimilate it in your body a lot faster so you are looking at a can of grapefruit juice a day; 60$ a month in grapefruit.

I've been on every combination and it's basically keeping me at base, and that's what I feel—right.... I've been on so many of them and I'm going on another one hopefully by the end of the month [Oct.98], I strongly believe that these medications kill viruses but they also have side effects, so they also kill a lot of good things as well. I'm at the point where I'm going on one more combination and if this doesn't … I'm sick of fucking doing this [taking drugs; having side effects]! … I'm going to try this new combination - cysteva plus 2 other ones.

Despite the buzz of optimism surrounding protease inhibitors and combination therapy, I witnessed considerable conflict and disillusionment set in among many HIV positive activists and other members of the HIV movement. Even when dramatic recoveries occurred, much uncertainty persisted among the HIV positive members of ACNS, who anticipated that the effectiveness of the new drugs would be temporary. Many members I spoke with expressed considerable anxiety around taking cocktail therapies, often fearing that the virus could mutate at any point and become resistant to their present drug therapy. When treatment resistance and failure did occur, they had to investigate other options for treatment. For some people I interviewed, their level of health was maintained but, like Larry, it was not straightforwardly improved. Experiencing considerable side effects, and sometimes temporary and uneven drug effectiveness, some of the HIV positive activists I interviewed at the time tried and eventually exhausted most of the options available to them and then had to resort to experimental treatments. During this time, many described how they felt "toxic" due to the sheer number of pills they were required to consume and the variety of drugs they had tried in their body; i.e., each new drug taking a period of time for the body to adjust. The inconsistent effects of these drugs and their complications agitated an already historically strained relationship these activists held with biomedical science and the health system.

The following ethnographic portraits of two important activists living in Nova Scotia who initially refused to take HAART, further sheds light on how ambivalent relationships formed between some of the AIDS activists and biomedicine.

2.2 Kent

I first met Kent in the early 1990s at a local fundraising event held for the NSPWA Coalition at the Roxbury nightclub, where he gave a rousing drag performance that brought the crowd to their feet in applause after singing a sultry torch song. Originally from the small island of Cape Breton, as a young gay man he had "escaped" to the urban centres of Edmonton and Toronto before finally returning to his home province of Nova Scotia. At the time we conducted our first interview, Kent was heading the home care program for the NSPWA coalition. In our interview in 1994 he began by telling me about his struggles to come to terms with his HIV status and the effect his diagnosis had on his interpersonal relationships.

> I had stopped paying bills … I was sleeping for days on end … I just generally didn't care anymore [for] probably about 2 years. I think I was in a stage of denial for a while … and for a long period of time after that, I really thought I was going to die soon; so I started to live that way. I cut off contact with my family that was the biggest thing. I didn't tell my family until 1990–1991....
>
> I didn't even tell people where I volunteered.... I didn't hide it from anyone; I just wasn't ready to talk about myself intimately … about my feelings with anyone which is an essential part of coming to terms with death. I told my partner … and he was the only one who knew and he had tested positive as well.
>
> It was very difficult because I also dealt with the fact that I probably gave it to him. We had a hard time dealing with that … we didn't care who gave it to who … that was the decision we had made … but it's still inside me … the suspicion that I had probably given it to him. For the first years that we had dealt with it we were dealing with it as a couple, and when I went to Toronto, Ted and I had in effect split up.... And when Ted got sick he came to Toronto at my request cause we had still kept in very close contact. So we picked up where we left off…. He lasted for two years.

During this interview, Kent recounted his tumultuous experience of taking AZT in the 1980s, at a time when its toxicity and efficacy were not fully known by scientists and clinicians and they were still experimenting with the dosages.

> When I did my first round of AIDS-related drugs, it was AZT at 1200 mg a day in the mid-80s. It was not really effective on its own. I mean all the studies show that it was 50/50. Fifty percent said it was effective; fifty percent said it was not. 1200 mg of AZT made me sicker than I had ever been in my life. It was like total poison. I stopped taking them. I mean I felt healthy until I started taking this drug and then all of a sudden I was as sick as a dog. This was 4 or 5 weeks into being on it.
>
> Anybody with a T-cell count less than 500, they were prescribing AZT for, and the lower your T-cell count was the more they were prescribing, basically. And mine was quite low. It was hovering around 200, and so they were giving me 1200 mgs a day. It made me totally sick. I quit taking them altogether, and about five or six months after that they cut that dose in half, universally, for everybody—universally to a maximum of 600 mg a day. (Sept., 1994)

This negative experience with AZT left an indelible scar on Kent's relationship to biomedicine, deeply embedding anxieties and distrust that affected Ken's refusal to adhere to future regiments.

Given the recognition of his leadership on the home-based care program at ACNS, Kent came to sit on the national board at the Canadian AIDS Treatment Information Exchange (CATIE) between 1996 and 1998 and helped to supervise my volunteer work at ACNS, which involved regularly updating the treatment files. In July of 1998, Kent told me that he was considering weighing the benefits of two treatment options he was given by the clinic:

> I've been given two options at the clinic—Crixivan, ddI and 3TC or the dual AZT and 3TC; so I have to choose one. Option A would be the optimum one with the protease inhibitor,

> however it's a tighter regime and I already told them that I have fears that I won't be complying, which is why I was reluctant to take the protease inhibitors before because it is essential that you comply with them. So I didn't want to start taking them, then not taking them; and have them [become] ineffective [due to viral mutation] when I *really* need them. The other option is to just take AZT-3TC combination.... That way I could take it in the morning and at night ... and that was it. It depends on how I can work it into my psychological framework ... into accepting them as part of my daily life.

When I spoke with Kent again later in November 1998, he told me that he went with the dual combination since his daily routine would be less affected by the regime. Kent was more concerned with maintaining "a certain quality of life over a certain viral load measurement," he said. I asked Kent if he thought the new drugs improved the well-being for PHAs and he said:

> It depends, if the drugs are providing you with a healthy quality of life ... that's great! If they are just diminishing viral load but you are sick all the time as a result of the drugs ... that's not so great—you are forsaking the quality of your life for the quantity and I would not do that for an instant. I would rather feel good and live a shorter life then feel sick all the time and live for years and years and years.

Kent claimed that he was not going to take a protease inhibitor combination until it was "absolutely necessary." He reasoned that the protease inhibitor would inevitably become resistant and then not work. Thus, he did not want to waste a potential future option. But his distrust of biomedical science, a legacy of his negative encounters with AZT, won out in his failure to adhere to this treatment regimen.

> [When] I took AZT and 3TC in combination. I really didn't give it too much of a chance because I felt pretty healthy ... I don't like the psychological ramifications of taking the drugs ... the fact that it was a reminder every day that I was living with this [HIV].

Kent was, in fact, highly conflicted in his view of the newer treatment options. Although there was a growing body of scientific evidence around clinical trials *efficacy* pertaining to new combination therapy, which he kept careful track of, their real world *effectiveness* was still highly uncertain for him. At the same time Kent was acutely aware of how his own negative experiences with previous generations of HIV therapy made him less receptive to the new class of ARVs, hindering his ability to adhere to treatment regiments:

> People who are newly diagnosed start off the game with much more hope than they have ever had previously ... they don't know the whole historical legacy of the drugs, [they] haven't been taught to be cynical and sceptical around drug therapies yet. So they might actually embrace them more openly. A lot of people who are newly diagnosed only read what they saw in the paper and it's all pretty upbeat. It's a magic bullet sort of stuff lately. So they might just assume that, well, OK I'm HIV positive but with these new drugs it's not going to be a problem; I still will get help and live a reasonably normal lifespan.... And that's not necessarily true ... they don't know the actual reality.
>
> We've had a lot of silver bullets over the past 12 or 13years, AZT-3TC and the rest of them. I mean protease inhibitors are a great drug...they are working for a lot of people ... they don't work for a lot of people.... We are just seeing now the effects of long-term usage ... people are now developing what they call "crix belly" and "crix hump" from Crixivan.

Although Kent had not taken protease inhibitors at the time of our interviews, when I asked him about how their existence had affected his perception of HIV as a chronic manageable illness, he responded as follows:

> I think that it's nice government speak and I think that they would like to have people believe that. But I've never known anybody to be cured of AIDS. I think asthma to be a chronic manageable illness because a lot of people have asthma ... and not many die of it. But as far as my knowledge ... everybody that has full blown AIDS dies ... protease inhibitors haven't been around long enough to see if they are going to change that or not. There is light at the end of the tunnel, even though I remain skeptical as to the efficacy. I can certainly see the results of it working now. I mean there is a much brighter hope for the future, even if these aren't "the ones" there might be a step two –"*the* ones!"

Despite his suspicions, in a later interview, Kent acknowledged the benefits arising from the release of protease inhibitors. He discussed the benefit in terms of the decrease in mortality rate:

> Because of the haste that they [protease inhibitors] were developed and released...I was skeptical; but I was also glad to see them and glad to hear of the promising things that they could do, because you heard this stuff before and it had always fallen through. I mean the results are astounding. You can go look at our book out there. It tells you how many of our members died, and the difference between last year and the year before that. Two years ago it was like 29 or 30 people. Last year it was like 5 or 6.

Kent's conflicted attitudes towards HAART and his adherence problems were not only shaped by his own negative experiences with AZT in the mid-1980s; but he explained to me that they grew out of what he was learning about from the struggles of others members of his community at ACNS while performing his role as the home-based care leader. He had learned that the daily lived experience of people taking HAART did not necessarily reflect the more straightforward picture of success painted in research findings, the news media, and government health policy. Indeed, the legacy of dissent toward biomedicine and health systems had nurtured a culture of resistance in community-based AIDS organizations, a climate which more generally stirred rebellious attitudes.

2.3 Nancy

At the time we were introduced in 1993, Nancy had assumed an important leadership role in the Black Outreach Project. Our common Caribbean background made for a fast friendship. In an initial phone conversation, I told her I was interested in meeting with her to conduct an interview. She wanted to be interviewed immediately, but when I mentioned that I would be unable to meet with her until I recovered from a cold (as it was my policy not to interview people living with HIV when I had a cold as I did not want to spread a cold virus to someone who was immune deficient), Nancy bluntly responded: "You take responsibility for yourself—if you can't come because you're not feeling well that's fine! But don't not come because you think I will get sick! Right now I'm taking care of my son who is sick. So you come over … I'm not that fragile."

Over the course of the interview Nancy recounted her journey that led to her HIV positive diagnosis:

> I got tested … my son and Peter got tested … and I was freaking cause I thought I was going to lose my whole family because we haven't had protected sex in years—before my child and after my child.
>
> Peter [Nancy's partner] and I had done a walk across Canada protesting uranium mining so that's how we ended up here in Nova Scotia … but through New Brunswick we had met lots of beautiful, heavy friends who had lived out in the bush and that's where I wanted to be, I wanted to be out in the bush.
>
> I also met a lot of native people. And I went out there and I called this native woman… right, who I had met brought the walk, and she was a friend and I thought…she said, "I knew you were coming," and I thought "bullshit"; I read those books too … right, those Lyn Andrews books, about these white women who write books about going into native culture, and native people telling them all this stuff. I told her, "I heard that one before," and she said, "Call me back when you decide not to be rude to me." So anyways, about two hours later she showed up at the door and she had sweet grass and a whole bunch of other stuff. She said I knew something heavy was coming down. "I want you to have courage, that is all that you need right now is courage," and "this is what you have to do." And she sends me all over Atlantic Canada to all these medicine women—to come to the sweats, right, and I'm saying, "You can't ask these women to do this. These women don't even know me. Why should they come hundreds of miles for this woman they don't even know? I have no money!" She says, "All you have to do is take them tobacco." So I did bring [tobacco] and then all of them came, and for three days and for three nights we fasted and sweat in the sweat lodge. It's built out of mud and trees. It's a prayer custom … it's a place where you are confined by mother earth, and it's completely dark and the rocks are gathered in a special way, in a very prayerful manner days before, and they are made to burn for 24 hours.
>
> Well the idea is praying—you see things, you know, because the people leading these sweats have to be medicine people … people who have had the training from childhood. So they go in and they pray. A lot of times I have gone through sweats and have seen things, lights, people, it's very dark. You're not supposed to see anything, but you see lights surrounding people, and things like that. Or you see spirits come in and sometimes you see spirits of avuncular ancestors or somebody else's. It's very hard to talk about it, this kind of stuff because people automatically believe, "Yeah she's crazy."
>
> So I came away from it knowing that I would be OK. I came away knowing that whatever direction my life was going to go in that I would be alright. It's more about having the courage to believe in myself, in my health and spirit. I don't know if I'm going to get AIDS and die. I don't think so. I don't believe HIV is the sole cause of AIDS to begin with; I believe it's a co-factor.
>
> I think it's a lifestyle. I think a lot of people who are HIV positive have also been leading very, very negative lifestyles; even through abuse in childhood or through manipulation from foreign power so that you have no good food or whatever. I don't believe that it's one specific thing but I do know nutrition is important and your mental health state is very important. (Nov. 1994)

Nancy's alternative perspectives on HIV aetiology and treatment were shaped by the activist networks she participated in prior to her work with the NSPWA; and it was further reinforced by the spirited culture of dissent of the HIV movement. For Nancy, illness was not something that resides in the physical body, but within "the spirit." Accordingly, to treat HIV she believed, one must "treat the spirit." She described her activism and political beliefs as being extremely leftist, and "anti-establishment." Biomedicine was to be rejected as "an instrument of white patriarchy" Nancy once declared during an interview. In terms of her own health, she only used alternative therapy, which she continued, following her HIV diagnosis in 1990:

> When I came back, I went to see one of the specialists here [in Halifax] who told me "Oh I guess you're anxious to get on AZT." So I said "No my T4-cell count is way too high. So I said, "What is it made out of? Maybe if you can tell me what it is made out of, I can get the natural ingredients and do it myself." She doesn't know. I said "You're prescribing shit to people and you don't know what is in it!" She says "Well the stats are what's important," and I said "Well fuck you and your stats." I was cussing so of course I got one hell of a reputation with the medical profession. My idea was to go completely alternative.
>
> With the first sweat, I was given an herb compound. An herb that kept coming up was akinesia fenugreek, alfalfa. My eating habits were looked at; the night that I left the sweat I had a dream. My ancestors kept coming to me, people I didn't even remember as being part of my tribe, per say, kept coming back. And there was this weird dream that kept saying hibiscus will heal you. And I thought now this is bullshit, this is complete crap because hibiscus is this plant that grows wild in my country [in the Caribbean], like the hedges. So I ignored it. I told a couple of friends. I told my husband that I had this dream and he went "Well, why don't you get some—just use it?" and I went to the North Shore to visit a good friend of mine and while I was there she brought out this book on hibiscus. [It] was one of the most potent blood cleansers in all of India, and I started to laugh. It was the same week that this had all happened, so I got some hibiscus flowers (that's what you're drinking), but I don't do it very often because I'm very healthy. It's only when I feel myself contracting a cold or something that I'll start getting all healthy and taking it and taking my akinesia. I also have a naturopathic doctor who lives in the Valley. She deals in herbs. Being with her is good because she has the same kind of basic philosophy that I have. (Nov. 1994)

Nancy's activism and her approach to caring for her body were intimately intertwined. And over the years of knowing her, her seemingly unfaltering positive health status justified her continued use of alternative therapies. The only anxiety she seemed to carry with respect to HIV related to her son:

> I always thought that I could manage this somehow. I feared for my son. I feared that he would be the one that would be infected. Now I fear that I won't be here to see him grow up, to have children. So my fear isn't about personally dying…. I lost my mother when I was three. Look at the shit I had to go through. Do I have to leave my son to that? So I get scared. (Nov. 1994)

During an interview in 1998, Nancy told me that her viral load was undetectable and her T-cells were very high. She claimed that her health had in no way deteriorated since 1994. As we walked with her son down the street in Halifax one day, in one of our many informal chats, she mentioned that she was still taking Echinacea and hibiscus and had also started taking evening primrose oil, which she complained about as being very costly. When I asked if there was any change in how she perceived HIV since we began our interviews, she responded:

> I was told by doctors that T-cell count was a measure of health … "this" was high, "this" was low. I could understand it from a scientific point of view … you know, but I could not relate to how this felt. I had no trust in it. It doesn't change my reality. I recognize and understand what medical professionals are saying about it, but [pauses] I believe, I perceive HIV as a tremendous lesson. Not as a terminal illness. Why have you entered my life?

I have something to learn from this. I personally will not die from this!! Maybe I'm in denial. Those who believe in protease need it. You have to believe in something!

Nancy's narrative is illustrative of both the existential questions and counter-narratives stirring within the walls of ACNS. Over time, ACNS began to offer, free of charge, an array of alternative therapeutic services aimed at increasing the immune systems of people living with HIV, including Swedish massage, reiki, reflexology, aura work, lymphatic massage, to information on nutrition, vitamin supplements, programs that promoted the benefits of exercise and lean-body mass, and spiritual retreat weekends. Promoted as complementary therapies, members living with HIV were encouraged by ACNS staff to try these alternative health services, to supplement conventional treatment regimes, and to help bolster their immune systems and help enhance their quality of life. There was even a designated room at ACNS where members were able to book an appointment with a particular practitioner. Although these therapies were highly valued by members of the community, as they helped to ease the illness experience by reducing stress, most positive members, unlike Nancy, did not depart from the hope that biomedicine would yield a breakthrough in treating or curing HIV and AIDS. As I discuss next, biomedical-coloured language characterized the dissent of this activist community as their embodied rebellions struggled with uncertain futures, amid anxiety and intense side-effects.

2.3.1 Bio-symbolism and Bio-sociality

I was diagnosed in 1985. The last T-cell count I had was in August of 1992. At that point it was 30; it was *really* low. It is probably really low right now if I have any at all…. I mean sometime I think about what that means that I am close [to death], you know, and I panic. But then I hear others talking about it and they have been around for a while, and are really low too. It gives me strength hearing their stories. They are survivors. (Les)

When I began interviewing AIDS activists living with HIV in early 1990s, many of the men and women I spoke with had lived through the experience of watching friends, lovers and partners die, all while encountering their own series of improvements and declines in their health status, along with treatment successes and failures. For many who were diagnosed in the 1980s, they had outlived their peers, thus resisting biomedical definitions based on their dwindling T-cell counts. "T-cell counts," as a biomedical measurement at the time, was considered a marker of decline in the health status of a person living with HIV. Yet some of the survivors I spoke with resisted the prognostic determinations that clinicians attached to T-cell counts; and they were deeply sceptical of the categorization of "full blown AIDS," which indicated the inevitable approach of sickness and death. Biomedical terminology helped to frame both the meanings of their journey with HIV at the same time as they questioned the realness of such measurements, challenging the interpretive authority of biomedicine to define the course of their illness.

The following quotations came from interviews I conducted with members of ACNS who described what it was like to live with HIV; even though I did not explicitly asked about their T-cell measurements, this biological marker reflected a crucial Leitmotif in their illness narratives.

> Fred: [My partner and my] T-cell counts are about the same. Last time I got it checked it was 140 and my partners was 130. That is low. Actually in the US if you are below 200 you are considered to have full blown AIDS. Here [in Canada] until you get an opportunistic infection (rare cancer or pneumonia) then you are not considered to have full blown AIDS. So [pauses] we aren't *there* yet. But some of our members we talk with, they go up and down a bit. I mean we have one friend who is at like 0 T-cells. He seems fine and is really living his life pretty normally, so it's hard to know what to make of the numbers sometimes. I try not to make too much of them, you know.
>
> Larry: I just got over the flu, really bad, and my T-cell count was 485 and it dropped to 192. In the US if you, if it drops below 200, you have full blown AIDS. But I have not had any opportunistic diseases, nothing that would indicate I would get full blown in the near future … T-cell count is something that we always mention when we see each other at the NSPWA [coalition], and we are just talking about our, our experience of this disease; it is like a way of telling people how you are feeling, and it's like a way of communicating how far you have to go, even though it's not really definite. I mean I have to go by how I feel and not just by those readings. The doctors don't know everything. [Larry]
>
> Tim: [when I was first diagnosed], I didn't know what [a T-cell count] was … you know, I knew that it was a specific white blood cell count and something to do with your immune system—you had 1200 if you were normal and at the 200 stage you had AIDS … so at that point I thought "Oh I'm going to be dying soon." But I've learned … I saw people with fluctuating T-cell counts where it would be 250 and then it would go up to 520 and anywhere in between … then I started to think that maybe I was not as close as I thought I was.
>
> Kent: I think my last count went down to 155 … because it had always hovered around 300. So that was a big jolt because that coupled with and an opportunistic infection would mean a diagnosis of full blown AIDS … but I felt completely healthy, I mean I really didn't worry about it too much because of my experience with so many other people. I mean I've seen people with virtually no T-cells live for 2 years and I have seen other people with less than 100 live for years and years.

In the era of monotherapy, prior to the release of protease inhibitors and combination therapy, conversations about "T-cell counts" not only led to contestation over the realness of biological measurements, but also these discussions helped produce the very social micro-fibres that tied together members through their experiences. As a universalistic biological metric, T-cell count narratives enabled PLWHA to create narratives that resonated with others experiences of living with HIV, invoking a particular kind of relatedness through blood. I repeatedly observed how the practise of sharing T-cell narratives in informal conversations imbued T-cells with social meaning that transcended biomedical notions of measurement; not only did these narratives question the definitiveness of "the numbers," but the very practise itself of sharing the narratives—discussing and questioning the limits of what T-cells can tell one about one's health—was part of how sociality was activated within this community. "T-cells" as a powerful metaphor allowed PLWHA to weave illness narratives, stories that spoke of their fears of death, their anxieties and hopes for the future, as well their struggles with biomedical interpretations of their bodies. Low T-cell counts certainly created intensity in the narratives that people shared. And despite uncertainties, T-cell count stories helped them to communicate their sense of how much time they might have left to live. The point here is that as a socially mobilized metaphor, "T-cell counts" carried with them an affective and interpretive force that created common resonances between members, even across very different background, sometimes bonding people across the spectrum of identity politics that sometimes swirled about the coalition offices. Despite, some political tensions between the gay men, women, members of the black community, indigenous people of first nations, sex workers, and people injecting and using drugs, I also witnessed how some conversations about T-cells, even if only for brief moments, appeared to melt away differences and competing political interests.

I am somewhat hesitant, though, to characterize the social boding created through T-cell talk as a manifestation of bio-sociality, a concept articulated by anthropologist Paul Rabinow. "Biosociality" (Rabinow 1999) can be defined as the formation of social relationships and identities around common genetic or biological conditions or afflictions. Undeniably, scientific terminologies and a common diagnosis underline the "persons living with HIV and AIDS" identity label as a form of personhood. But there were inherent tensions I observed in such "T-cell talk," to borrow the words of Robert Ariss and Gary Dowsett (1997); for the narrators work to unsettle the epistemological claims of biomedicine. T-cell talk, as a narrative of self-determination and resistance, allowed people living with HIV to deconstruct the biomedical narrative of precision and exactitude. We may then think of T-cell talk as a form of critical exegesis that exemplifies a begrudged biosociality, a sort of friction embodied in their relationships to biomedicine. While activists living with HIV re-employed T-cells as a metaphor that was rich with meaning and resonant with the experiences of others, at the same time it accented the uniqueness of one's bodily-being as resisting scientific classification. Putting it another way, they simultaneously appeal to a cellular-level universalism at the same time as they oppose a cellular reductionism of their illness experience, raising ontological questions about T-cells based on their daily lived reality with HIV.

Although there continued to be a lot of T-cell talk following the release of combination therapy in 1996, the meanings and emotions expressed around T-cell counts changed dramatically with the introduction of the new measurement referred to as "viral load," which measured the number of HIV particles per ml.

> Kyle: back in the 80s early 90s I expected that what happened to my partner would most certainly happen to me. His T-cells were reduced to 4, and then I slowly watched him disappear and die. [A declining] T-cell count meant death to me, and back then I waited for my count to drop as Leo's had. Today, with viral load testing and as well as a growing arsenal of new protease inhibitors, I still pay too much attention to the numbers; but they are not as much a source of fear as before. Those readings aren't, well, fixed.

And Rick, a long-term survivor of 14 years similarly discussed this change in meaning:

> The T-cell count used to be the end all, I mean you ran home and said "my T-cell count was down to 304" and you were really scared ... and now you think – who cares? It's not really important anymore. The emphasis is on the viral load now. Even though that is where the emphasis is, that doesn't really mean that much to me now. It fluctuates. But it is also how

> I feel … and even though I've had a count of 220 and a count of 260 and had a viral load of 18,000 and then 226,000 … I feel the same. If my body is telling me that I don't feel well … that's what I'm listening to … I don't listen to viral load and to T-cell count and all that crap.

As these narrative suggest, protease inhibitors and the introduction of viral load measurement—which was considered to offer a much more reliable measure of HIV-related illness progression— did not eliminate uncertainty in their illness experience. Viral load, in fact, introduced greater uncertainty into the process of tracking the progress of HIV for clinicians and the activists alike. The larger looming narrative of decline previously expressed in the era monotherapy through T-cell counts, were replaced with viral load talk, which furnished narratives with multiple climaxes and denouements, and unresolved conclusions. Viral load, considered in biomedical science as more precise given the smaller microbiological units it represented compared to T-cells, was found to be a much more fluctuating type of measurement.

Between 1996 and 1998, the earlier fears and anxieties around the inevitability of death I had encountered were transformed to frustration, uncertainty and anxiety with regards to side effects from the new drugs, as portrayed in their viral load narratives. Members also began taking part in clinical trials with experimental drugs as they began to run out of treatment options. I was struck by the dialogue used to describe their treatment experiences. It became increasingly laden with medical terms, drug names, and clinical descriptions of side effects. Indeed biomedical language had begun to colour the illness narratives shared between PLWHA much more noticeably than when I had begun my study in the early 1990s. Although the dialogue between these men and women superficially appeared to echo the language of biomedicine, this "medical creole" (Ariss and Dowsett 1997), however, accomplished a different end for these activists by challenging biomedical authority. The knowledge they were able to express in their talk was steeped in experiential knowledge rather than medical training. In other words, it was individual experience that underscored the epistemological claims in their counter narratives.

> I tried to get it [a T-cell count taken] on my own; you insist on it as much as you can if you've had it done one month ago … they are not going to do it. Same with viral load … there has to be some reason for it … there has to be some crisis before it is done. I should be able to go in and say, "Yes, it is time now! I want my viral load done! I want that done now!" I mean I know my health. I am living with this. I can judge when I need my viral load taken, even when the doctors don't think I need it.

As illustrated in the narratives of this section, some HIV positive activists, particularly long-term survivors, came to trust their bodily experiences over the technical measurements of their health. Because the "medical creole" and counter narratives I encountered in my fieldwork were expressed in the safety of the coalition environment or in members' homes, they can be considered as a locally-situated linguistic form—that is, a "dialect" which only this community of activists can claim and assert. While members and medical professionals use the same terms such as viral load or T-cell counts, only the daily lived experiences with the illness can breathe meaning and a sense of knowing into these measurements. At the same time, the growing density of biomedical language reflects the further entanglement of activism in biomedical regimes.

2.4 The Tyranny of Drug Regiments

Protease inhibitors brought about tremendous transformations in health as well as uncertainty and challenges around side-effects. Combination therapy at the time of my study in the later 1990s also brought extremely demanding treatment regiments that many of the activists considered to be highly intrusive in their everyday lives.

Idioms of death were replaced with outbursts of frustration as activists attempted to adhere to their medication regiments. Numerous pills and beepers that marked daily life into temporal intervals not only served as a continual reminder of the illness but of the entanglement of their lives with biomedical authority and technologies. Many of the activists spoke of their own rebellious desires toward the disciplining effects of their treatment regiments.

> Tim: well I don't have a little clinic one [beeper], but I have one of my own you know … and it drives me crazy. So, it still goes off at 11 o'clock … and some nights the fucking things [pills] can just stay in the fridge … they can stay there as far as I'm concerned. Whether it's a beeper or a handful of pills or whatever it is. It's a fucking reminder that you are HIV positive.
>
> Rick: the beeper makes me angry. I hate it when it goes off, I want to break it. It reminds me of my physical condition. Well, picture your alarm going off three times every day … I have to stay up, I may be dropping with sleep, but I have to stay up 'til close to midnight to take them or else turn the beeper off which means it's not going off in the morning … so, I can't turn it off. It rules my life so I take it wherever I go and its load. You know you are at a meeting and the damn thing goes off.
>
> Les: I think that's one of the biggest challenges in dealing with all those drugs is how you manage your social life. Some of these drugs you have to diet, before eating, an hour before taking the drugs and other drugs you have to eat a little something with times you take them your drug times may not correspond to mealtimes and it is a real pain in the ass sometimes.
>
> Larry: every eight hours, some are every six hours, some have to be taken with food … others don't. Sometimes I set my dam clock and say to myself, "To hell with it, my sleep is more important!" I keep on as strict a regiment as I can, without letting it overtake my daily routine. My medication in the morning is done with food. Suppertime … if I'm out somewhere having supper at a friend's place … if I don't have my medication, it's not a big thing. I'll have two soda crackers or what not and have them when I get home. I won't wake up in the middle of the night if I feel I really need the sleep.
>
> I don't know how to describe it … it's a daily routine and it's like … sometimes I just wish I could biff the fucking bottles out of the apartment … I mean I know people who would say, well, you are lucky you live in Canada … you have access to all these drugs … and I tell them you try them! I just wish I could wake up one morning and say I don't have to swallow these pills. That's unrealistic for me night now.

Sam described himself as having a "very structured" and organized personality. I sometime jokingly commented on how "compulsively neat" his office was always kept. Quality of life, according to Sam, was influenced by his ability to have a structured daily routine. Due to the unpredictable nature of the drugs he was taking, his daily routine had continually to bend to accommodate his drug regime:

> [E]specially with ritonavir, you can eat next to nothing without it upsetting you … I was down to bananas and toast at one point … that's all I could eat and then with Nelfinavir, I could eat anything and then you are starving …you want to eat everything. So you are trying to get a plan for your life and you really can't … different side effects … I was lactose intolerant for a while … I am not now.... same with exercise. You may get into a regime that you want to stick with, and then you are not feeling well so you have to stop. Some drugs are very debilitating and you can't do it [exercise] because of diarrhoea or whatever other side effects … and then the next drug you are fine again … so you get back in that regiment. It's just … there's no consistency!!
>
> The people that I am with … they have to understand that I have to take pills … I may not want to eat at 4:00, but I have to … and I don't want to eat at 8:00 in the morning. I've always liked to eat when I felt like eating. I can't do that because my drugs have to be taken with food. So, unless I'm going out somewhere, if I'm going to be there around midnight … I have to excuse myself and go into a corner and eat something and take pills. I have to watch the time and plan!

As a gifted artist, Sam lived by himself in an apartment complex. During one of our interviews, he told me that he lacked the emotional support of close friends since he left Toronto and shared how this affected his daily routine.

> I don't have a regular friend to watch me. I've had to take care of myself. [Taking medication] three times a day is really difficult, plus I take Septra for thrush, ganciclovir for CMV, Imodium® for diarrhoea, Stemetil for nausea. I take stuff for itch for hiving cause it is very uncomfortable. If I sat on my butt at home I would have no problem … but you know I like to be active and sometimes I do miss a dose or forget.

According to members of ACNS I interviewed, they frequently complained that clinicians focussed on the physical and biological nature of their side effects but did not ask them how these side effects actually impacted on their daily lives as social beings. Demanding treatment regiments dominated over social meanings. But at the same time, as treatment regiments enacted biomedical hegemonies, inflaming the bodies of these activists into sites of rebellion against biomedical tyranny, the field of experimental drugs offered fertile terrain for reimaging and enacted new forms of AIDS activism.

2.5 Involvement in Clinical Trials

In the summer of 1998, I was contacted by Rick, the head of the organizing committee for a support group called the Positive Action Group. This support group, consisting of 30 HIV positive members at the time, planned a variety of social activities that ran independently of ACNS health programs. Rick described the group as "just like a normal group of friends who do things together but don't sit around and talk about HIV or AIDS." As I came to know the members of the support group well I learned how The Positive Action Group functioned to ease the experience of living with HIV and AIDS. Rick explained that the support group created a space in which

PHAs felt safe, understood, and not judged. Nevertheless, over the coming years this safe space increasingly filled with the echoes of frustration around the release of new drugs, the demanding treatment regimes, and their participation in clinical trials.

In the first few months of my ethnographic research with the Positive Action Group, I conducted focus groups with members of their organizing committee. Together we identified key issues in the development of a qualitative interview guide that explored the concerns of the support group. In particular, I was requested by Kent (mentioned earlier in this chapter) to interview the support group members about their treatment experiences and their growing involvement in clinical trials.

2.6 A Clinical Trials Community

> Rick: The drugs I'm taking now are all trials …I think they [the clinicians] are running out of options … The one I was taking before now was saquinavir and ddI, the hard one; it's like a big wafer. The first reaction was good—18,000 was my viral load which is marvellous compared to where it was … the next time it was back up. Crixivan wasn't doing anything for me … my viral load zoomed up to 156,000 on Crixivan, 3TC and d4T. nelfinavir I got the same story … there aren't many [combinations] left.

Most participants regarded ARVs that were still at the clinical trial phase as viable treatment options, at a moment of time when dosages and effectiveness for approved medications were still being determined by clinical scientists. In other words, there was a blurring in distinction between approved and experimental drugs, as members were in some sense also experimenting with new combinations with their clinician to discover the right combination that worked. Moreover, new clinical trials were particularly important for members like Rick who had tried and exhausted all other approved treatment options. Participants sometimes perceived these experimental medicines as being no more or less predictable or effective than approved drug regimes. Most of the support group members discussed their first hand experiences with clinical trials conducted at the infectious disease clinic in Halifax, located in the Dixon Centre of Dalhousie Medical School. Thus, clinical trials participation formed a shared experience of this group. Although not every HIV positive member accessing services at ACNS participated in clinical trials, a vibrant and savvy clinical trials community emerged in this small urban centre of eastern Canada.

One member of this trials community was Tanya who was actively involved with ACNS as one who both received and provided health services. She served as a peer counsellor and provided support group facilitation for her peers. Having formerly worked as a health care professional for many years, and having obtained an MA in a health-related discipline, she was an ideal choice as the representative of ACNS on the advisory board for the Canadian HIV Trials Network (CTN). Compared to other mostly gay male members of the support group, Tanya's diagnosis in 1992 was recent. She did, however, have considerable experimental treatment experience including her participation in an interferon clinical trial.[2] Tanya discussed her experiences of grave disappointment with the clinical trial process which precipitated her eventual involvement with the CTN advisory board as a community activist:

> So I went on that trial [interferon] and I got sicker and sicker … and I called the doctors more than ever because of the trial … and I'm going in there and I'm telling them; they never took any of the cues from me. You know, I'm going in there and I'm saying, 'I'm short of breath, I'm really feeling terrible.' They went through their little routines, they asked the questions, they totally ignored the signals … and *I was not giving intellectual signals, I was giving them emotional signals* and trying to tell them I felt terrible. I had diarrhoea from one drug so then we changed over to the other one … and they went through all the mechanical things, like checking for salmonella and all that … but they never dealt with the fact that I was … my hair was falling out all kinds of things were going on. Finally I went in for one of these routine tests. I mean you have an interview with a nurse, you talk about things. I was saying, "I'm short of breath, I'm having trouble breathing." I felt terrible, and he [the doctor] wanted to palpate my abdomen … and I'm saying I find it difficult to lie down, and these buggers aren't paying attention to what you say. They just go on their back and I got up and I went home and called and made an appointment with my family doctor.
>
> I went and I said, "I think I'm dying." I was just desperate and I never made a lot of visits to my family doctor. I told my family doctor the same things I had told the other guy … and the family doctor had the skill to look at the bigger picture instead of focussing on the HIV … he looked at the whole thing and listened to what I was saying … what was happening was that my thyroid had been hyper … so the family doctor gave me a drug that started blocking the hormone.
>
> Meantime, I go back to the clinic for the drug trial … I was still taking things … I told them what had happened … they never said anything to me like, "Tanya, we should have picked this up!" And I got angry cause when I came away I thought, why did somebody not sit down and talk to me about and make me realize that I was poorly attended to? I had been "looked" at by the attendants, but poorly attended to … cause I slipped right through!

Paralleling AIDS activism in the USA, as described by Stephen Epstein (1996), HIV-related activism in Canada, which was animated through networks of dynamic "patient-advocates," succeeded in making inroads into the clinical trials regulatory environment, a domain traditionally under the jurisdiction of biomedicine. Paltiel and Stinnet (1996) discuss how AIDS activists came to challenge and even regulate the authority of clinicians at this time. Tanya, as a result of her frustration and disappointment during her participation in an interferon clinical trial, became the regional representative for the CTN advisory board. This advisory board was designed to oversee the ethical considerations of clinical trials and to advance the interests of participants undergoing clinical trials. One of their main objectives was to review and revise consent forms for drug trial participants. Tanya explained:

> In the trials network committee, we are pushing real hard that there'd be a continuation if you are on an experimental drug, and you finish the trial and the drug is waiting to come on to the provincial formulary, [when] it is legal for sale in Nova Scotia (as opposed to Health Canada saying it is legal for use in Canada). You've just taken a fantastic drug that has done really well for you; the chances are that you will be completely cut off, because, from the time the trial finishes to the time it actually gets on to the market in Nova Scotia, (which is the only time you can write a prescription and get it), it could be quite a time frame. It could

[2] Interferon is an immune strengthening drug that mimics a substance that white blood cells make.

be six months, which in HIV terms might be too long for me—I'd be dead. So that's why when somebody enrols in a trial we try to get it written into every one of the agreements [consent forms]—that if the PHA wishes to continue the drug, it is provided by the company until such time as it gets on the formulary.

Many drugs like saquinavir and indinavir … if you did well on the trial, and now the trial is finished you can continue with that drug cause it's already on the formulary and it is already a registered drug. But some of these new drugs are not. So they can be on hiatus … a time that you were not able to access that drug. Not every drug company will put its drugs on expanded access.

If you are person X, who knows of a drug that is not yet available … but he is not looking at being involved in trials at all… Because the drug is "in trials" … he is not eligible for them, presumably. So while the trial is going on … but it is in Toronto. It's not here … we only have a tiny few … he knows of that drug, he knows that it might be good for him so the only way to get it is through the doctor making an argument with the drug company to provide that drug through compassionate release. It's not out on the market yet, it's not freely available, but it's a last hope for somebody.

It was through compassionate release that Nadine was able to obtain a drug which enabled her to leave palliative care:

They had a new pharmacist come in from down the States from Boston … She had suggested that I go on what she had tried on people in the States … she was putting them on half dosages … so we tried a combination of half dosages. Legally, I shouldn't have been on it because my T-cell count wasn't in the criteria … I was so advanced. The way I understand it, the clinic gets the drugs and the government pays for them but they have to follow the criteria … I was too far gone, so I hounded and hounded them and got it on compassionate release so I went on what I'm still on it now … saquinavir, ritonavir and d4T.

In the autumn of 1998, Les had begun treatment with *Vistide*—a drug used to treat CMV that was being tested in the USA. He was granted approval for this drug through compassionate release. Les shard with me the extensive regiment to which he adhered:

To take that drug [Vistide] it is very, very toxic … I have to prepare hours before I go into the hospital. It usually takes a day to administer the drug through IV. I have to prepare before I go in the hospital by taking medications to prevent side effects … then I go into the hospital, I usually get two litres of saline to flush my veins before they start pumping in the drugs. I probably take 40 pills a day and the IV treatment is once every three weeks now.

Paltiel and Stinnet maintain that the increase in regulatory power enacted by AIDS coalitions produced a shift from "a strictly scientific focus to a more consumer-centred orientation" (1996: 1054). The scientific goals of clinical research were re-focused, through the growing influence of advocacy groups in the CTN, around the wellbeing of the individual patient, thus rendering more flexible regulations on clinical trials access. Consequently, HIV trials increasingly came to serve the needs of consumers, particularly those who had exhausted other pharmaceutical options on approved formularies. Les, who had also served on the CTN advisory board, recounts his reason for getting involved with clinical trials while telling of his ability to assert his "lay expertise" (Epstein 1995):

I was on the CTN advisory team and I knew what the trials were even before they were approved. We discussed approving them. So very often when they were approved, (that's probably about a year from the time they were presented until they were approved) … then

> I would assess the exclusion–inclusion criteria to determine whether or not I could [take the drugs] and I would talk to my doctor about that. I have a very good relationship with the clinic if I go to [names doctor] and say I need this and I have this condition … he will take my word very often. If I call up and say I want to switch drugs, very often there is little debate … and he'll do that.

Sam, eventually becoming a project coordinator at ACNS and after having read the treatment update files, decided he too would get involved in a clinical trial:

> I read about it [evening primrose oil study], I asked [the clinic] if I could be involved in it … because I had nothing to lose at that point … my T-cells were rapidly declining … here was maybe a chance to bring them back up. I didn't know much about viral load back then … when the viral load was taken here it had to be shipped to Vancouver to be read … so we didn't even have the equipment to read viral load … so I wanted to give it a shot.

The scientific goals of clinical trials are to produce data that would permit the evaluation of drug efficacy. Given the "consumeristic" approach taken by the trials community in Halifax, who were looking for new therapeutic options, the "scientific" goal of clinical trials often became secondary to them. ACNS members often chose not to adhere to clinical trial regimes when they perceived that there was no longer of benefit. When Tim became involved in his first clinical trial in 1994, he had very low expectations of what to expect in terms of efficacy. He evaluated the trial (1994) in which he participated as being ineffective:

> July, 25 1993,I was diagnosed as positive … shortly thereafter, I joined a clinical trial. It was one injection of interferon three times a week … the clinic suggested it, I was thinking that AZT was probably the better of the two. The trial wasn't that important. I personally felt guilty by saying no so I said "Yes." I felt pressured … that I should somehow be doing something to help other people … I had no side effects but there weren't any significant changes … I dropped out. I didn't see any benefit to it … no physiological changes.

Tim also expressed anger, frustration and resentment with the clinic as well as his continually changing treatment regime. He finally decided to go off all medications:

> "That's expensive!" That's your experience at the clinic: "We give you these drugs, you have to take them because they cost money … and if you don't take them, you are taking them away from other people who will take them"—guilt! [After the interferon trial], I continued with AZT … when 3TC was approved I was put on that … I was then switched to a triple combination of saquinavir, ritonavir and d4T … I take I5 pills, 7 in the morning and 8 in the evening. I'm not taking anything right now. Summer came and I had had enough of the numb lips, and the diarrhoea and the aches and the pain and all that shit … and the rigidity of the regime.

After his first experience with a clinical trial, when approached by the clinic on participating in another trial Tim decided not to become involved:

> I turned it down … because I don't like to take pills. I'm not a very good person as far as pills go. Because the follow-up is so rigid, and my time commitment here [at ACNS] and my time commitment to other things … I just don't have the time.

Taking a drug holiday was a common occurrence among the community of activists I interacted with. The following three quotations illustrate the kind of explanations individuals provided for temporarily abandoning their treatment regiments:

> Stan: I may stop taking any medication except for [the ones that prevent opportunistic infections]. I mean it comes down to quality versus quantity. You know I've worked too hard to stay fit to go around with fatty deposits [from Crixivan].
>
> I've gone on drug holidays because you become so toxic … and you can't face them anymore … it's a constant reminder … that you are taking AIDS medication, that you are taking all these things and you don't know what they are doing to you … you really want to take them … but you just wonder how much damage it's doing to other things …you could die of kidney failure.
>
> Larry: sometimes I go off medication without telling them. You just get pissed off, your popping 20, 25 pills a day … and it's a full time job if you had to sit down and monitor your pills.
>
> Tanya: after that drug trial [interferon], I went off it … I said I need a drug holiday … and I went off everything 8 or 9 months until I had some low T-cells … I actually dipped below 200 … then I went on AZT 3TC until June of 98. I'm actually not taking anything right now.
>
> In June of this year I suddenly got detectible … I was 81,000, [viral load] then 6 weeks later 25,000 … that's why now I've stopped the drugs I've been on … cause now I'm waiting to go on a regime of two protease inhibitors … I'm going away this weekend Thanks Giving] and I'm going to start it after I come back.

There were only three people I interviewed who had never (or only rarely) deviated from their treatment regiments. They maintained throughout the interview that biomedicine was their best route to slowing the progression of the virus.

> Rick: I've never considered it [drug holiday] … I shouldn't say I've not considered
>
> It, cause every day I swear at them … I am really bad at taking pills … not bad … I follow the regime, I have a beeper. They make me gag mostly.
>
> Kyle: I have no problem adhering to my medication schedule, and the hospital visits and all the blood work that is necessary are just that—necessary! I have always tolerated drugs such as AZT very well.
>
> Sam: If I don't take ganciclovir and then I get CMV and go blind that's pretty good incentive to take your pills. So, I don't even think of it. It's just part of my life and I just do it.

Larry was informed of a Cysteva and ddI trial by the clinic in October 1998. He decided that he would get involved despite the numerous failures he had already encountered with clinical trials in the past. Larry had run out of options.

> They [the clinicians] told me about the trial [Cysteva]. When the medication isn't doing what it is supposed to be doing … they usually suggest that you go on something else … whatever is available. I've been on all the NDA approved cocktails.
>
> I have no other options … and realistically speaking, in my mind I don't think it's going to do much for me … because I've been on so many combinations … I'm doing it for other people … they might find something in my chemistry that will help another individual.

Larry maintains that altruism was a critical factor that influenced his decision to become involved with clinical trials. As it was explained to me, clinicians frequently encouraged members of the HIV movement who were living with AIDS to help in the struggle to find effective treatments. This rationale resonated well with the politically engaged trial community. Already committed to being "agents of social action," they believed that their actions as individuals could potentially improve conditions of life for others. Kyle and Sam also discussed altruism as a key consideration for becoming involved in clinical trials:

> Kyle: I was asked by the clinic doctor if I would like to participate in a drug trial (d4T, 3TC and 141 W94 which is amprenovir), and I said, "Yes I would" … I guess. Because I was sitting by for years doing nothing, not being part of the struggle … I guess this is my way of making a contribution … also at the same time … I think in the back of my mind … it provided me with an opportunity to get on a cocktail. I had never been on a cocktail before.
>
> Sam: when I was reading about it [evening primrose oil phase one trial, 19951, it was talked about glowingly . . . because when they talked about killing HIV in the test tube … I said I would give it a try. I was sort of hoping that something would come out of Nova Scotia … some kind of miracle. It was very disappointing, but I just said, OK, it didn't work, what is next.

Despite the many disappointments expressed in the stories of ACNS members and activists who experienced little or no direct benefit from their participation, some continued to get involved in clinical trials. At times I wondered why some members had a fundamental distrust of "the clinic" while others were avid supporters—why was there such a split in attitudes? When I posed this question to Tanya, she responded:

> You know there are a lot of people who get a jolly out of having the attention around a trial … cause you go in very regularly, right … you' re given attention.... if you are that kind of personality … for me that doesn't work … for me that doesn't work. I don't need that kind of attention I'd rather go elsewhere for attention. It's very personalized [the clinic encounter] "How are you doing Robert?" … you get the chance to sit down and talk about yourself. They're getting one-on-one attention paid to them. My need from them is to be dealt with compassionately or respectfully but maximizing the benefit for me.

At the same time, Tanya acknowledged that she had benefited from those who engaged in clinical trial over the years:

> I'm not a front-runner here … there's people out ahead of me … and I am very happy they are there … because here is the big kick-off for me. They have given me information by going into trials and doing those types of things … that has allowed me to feel quite comfortable this number of years down the road … so I'm very happy and very grateful that other people are out there ahead of me … and I'm sort of the second wind coming out behind them … benefiting.

Tanya maintained a suspicion, however, that the supposed "scientific focus" of the clinicians concealed a broader commercial agenda on the part of pharmaceutical companies. Although she engaged in many social justice activities, advocating for the rights of people living with HIV and AIDS at the CTN advisory board, Tanya did not believe that subjecting one's body to clinical trials was a viable way to take action for the greater good of PHAs.

> I wouldn't go into a trial 'for the greater king of man' … I'm not about to put my body out and have it … so somebody can write another paper … I'm more selective about what happens to me and my body … I mean some of these trials that are coming up are scary stuff like lumbar punctures.

It's sort of like the salesman situation they're in … they've got clinical trials running that they need candidates for … and if you are selling a product; say you are a used car salesman and you've got two cars and there is a better mark-up on one … you'd much rather get rid of that one off your lot, then you promote it. So, I think that it's all done in the name of your best interest at heart, but there's the inclination to want to fill the numbers, getting research finding, write papers, all wrapped up with it.

Nowadays, there are so many different options to be offered, so if people justify it as doing it for the good of others.... Hopefully people are well informed, and that's the hard part. They are now corning up with a lot of trials that involve biopsies of lymph nodes … and the latest ones we are seeing involve the spinal fluids. Now do you want to go and have lumbar punctures? I'm thinking … oh my god … I just don't have the guts to do that!

In a subsequent interview, Tanya's explained that her experiences with clinical trials helped her to realize the broader agenda of clinicians. As an active member of CTN advisory board, she helped to protect the interests of PLWHA from the "business of pharmaceutical industry." Tanya cited the following experience as having opened her eyes to the potential compromise of a patient's well-being for the benefit of clinical research pursuits:

I had been talking to the clinic, "What about protease?" And they said "You're fine on what you have and we're not touching anything." Then they asked me into a drug trial that was double protease and a non-nucleoside.... Why is it they are telling me that I'm not eligible for protease under normal circumstances … so why am I suddenly eligible to do a drug trial? Well that is the problem with drug trials; they're kind of rattling the cages to find clientele.

Les, who became the executive director of ACNS, described his ambivalent relationship with biomedicine. On one hand, he needed more options; on the other, he distrusted the agenda of the pharmaceutical industry.

The current drugs I'm on are nelfinavir, and 50 92 V [anti-inflammatory drug to treat herpes zoster] and a couple of prophylactic drugs. I'm on Vistide which is a drug currently access through the emergency releases plan because it is not available in Canada for CMV retinitis. I would argue that the medical profession sometimes is not necessarily prolonging life … I mean I would argue that sometimes they are only interested in prolonging misery just to test their products or test their scientific skills manipulating people's misery.

Prior to my starting Crixivan in late 95 … I was not feeling well and certainly that product did do wonders for me. I was on a triple combination of Crixivan, 3TC and ddI … and I did do very well. I felt much better for a year and a half to 2 years but then I started to fail that combination. From there I have moved on to several other combinations and now the drugs that I am on are only accessible through the emergency drug release plan … because all the approved drugs I've failed … I'm running out of options.

My body has been used as a laboratory for a very long time now. I choose to do that … I choose to engage in drug trials … I choose to let pharmaceutical companies test drugs on my body. It has nothing to do with being altruistic. Many PHAs don't get involved in drug trials to help "the cause"; or anything like that … hopefully they will have some effect … probably [they get involved] because there is nothing else there.

While conducting the provincial needs assessment, as discussed in the first chapter, I witnessed how pharmaceutical companies did in fact target HIV CBOs. At that time, major drug corporations hired full-time public relations employees to work with HIV coalitions in Nova Scotia. For example, one day I was introduced to a representative from a leading pharmaceutical company during one of her visits in the small town of Sydney, Nova Scotia. She was soliciting AIDS service organizations throughout Nova Scotia for HIV drug trial participants. The AIDS coalition in Cape Breton I was visiting at the time had already received a number of visits from her and jokingly called her "the cheerleader" given her strikingly quaffed hair and unrelenting cheery disposition, even amid rather grave matters.

That day she arrived in her tan business suit driving a matching tan Cadillac she had rented. It was a rather striking scene to see such affluence and formality paraded in Sydney, a small working class town which held some of the highest unemployment rates (over 30 % then) in the country. She began the conversation with us by talking of a "new cocktail trial" that had just begun enrolling patients. The pharmaceutical representative then asked me if "the clients" I worked with knew of this trial. She began to speak glowingly of the promising results that the trial had to offer. I then raised the concern that many of the members at the CBO would likely not be eligible for the new trial, because most members who were injecting drugs were co-positive for hepatitis C. In regions like Cape Breton, where HIV and hepatitis infections spread rapidly among people injecting drugs (Lior et al. 1998); most ARVs at the time could not be offered to them given the damaging effects of the drugs on the liver, a fact which one of the outreach managers reminded the drug representative, in a sharp tone. To this, the representative responded by saying that "they" could fly in one of "their IDU specialists" to meet with "our clients." (I noticed some of the staff of the organization quietly cringed each time she said "clients.")

Throughout our conversation, the representative talked about the numerous conferences "their specialist" had been able to attend across Canada and the USA in the last month, trying to establish his credibility as an expert. She reminded us that money was no object to this company in being able to help the PHA community. They could fly in any of "their people" for a retreat weekend with "our IDUs" if we so requested. The director of the coalition suggested an alternative plan to the costliness of flying in an expert, which would involve setting up a support group for people who inject drugs who were confronting struggles to live positively with HIV and hepatitis C. This program could provide a source of much needed honoraria to "our members," he added. The drug representative was less than cheery at this suggestion and persisted in maintaining the importance of flying in one of their specialists.

As some of the group challenged her, the drug representative then began to discuss her volunteer work with people with AIDS to show us how genuinely committed to caring about people she was. However, the staff at the coalition were not convinced and felt it was clear that her priority was to promote the company futures sales over advancing the present well-being of their members. Flying in a specialist from BC to spend a few hours at a cost of thousands of dollars was clearly less helpful to members and only served the promotional interests of their company. The AIDS coalition staff stood firm before the pharmaceutical representative in their assertion that the money would be better spent if it were given to sustain programs that offered psychosocial support year round rather than for a few brief hours.

***

The type of treatment narratives presented in this chapter, although suggesting a tendency toward individualized and consumeristic orientations, portray more than solely internalized personal struggles. The re-telling and sharing of these kinds of stories in the safe spaces that activists created for themselves can be conceptualized as *becoming* political, fomenting dissenting perspectives that challenge, while also relying upon, scientific interpretations and measurements of the body. In other words, they inherently reach outwardly, affecting social connections between members of the movement living with HIV and AIDS. Their narratives of uncertainty and frustration over the correct dosages and combinations of new HIV treatment advancements during this historical moment reflected the entanglement of an activist community in an experimental terrain that germinated new forms of dissent, creating emotionally deep yet ambivalent connections between activism and biomedical science. Bodily encounters with the unpredictable and inconsistent effects of these drugs formed the existential ground on which activists generated counter-knowledges to mobilize their position in creating new ethical conditions within clinical trials regulatory environments. Previously, CTN regulatory officials formulated clinical trials guidelines from within their protected citadel of scientific distance and detachment, removed from the lived experiences of those participating in the clinical trials. However, with the inclusion of people living with HIV on advisory boards, the intimate knowledge produced through embodied conflicts with pharmaceutical substances and trials scientists transformed this policy terrain, redefining the knowledge that counts by grounding ethical decision making in lived realties that mattered from the perspective of quality of life.

References

Ariss, R. M., & Dowsett, G. W. (1997). *Against death: The practise of living with AIDS* (Vol. 5). New York:Psychology Press.

Epstein, S. (1995). The construction of lay expertise: AIDS activism and the forging of credibility in the reform of clinical trials. *Science, Technology & Human Values, 20*(4), 408–437.

Epstein, S. (1996). *Impure science: AIDS, activism, and the politics of knowledge* (Vol. 7). Berkeley: University of California Press.

Kempf, D. J., Marsh, K. C., Denissen, J. F., McDonald, E., Vasavanonda, S., Flentge, C. A., et al. (1995). ABT-538 is a potent inhibitor of human immunodeficiency virus protease and has high oral bioavailability in humans. *Proceedings of the National Academy of Sciences, 92*(7), 2484–2488.

Lior, L., Stratton, E., & Archibald, C. P., et al. (1998). *Eastern Region Project: Seroprevalence of HIV, HBV, and HCV viruses and high risk behaviours among IDU and sexual partners of IDU*. Slide presentation, Health Canada.

Paltiel, D. A., & Stinnet, A. A. (1996). AIDS. In B. Spiker (Ed.), *Quality of life and pharmacoeconomics in clinical trials* (pp. 1053–1060). Philadelphia: Lippincott-Raven.

Rabinow, P. (1999). From sociobiology to biosociality. In *The science studies reader* (p. 407). New York: Routledge.

Part II
India: Techno-Bureaucratization

Chapter 3
Geographies of Intervention

Abstract Based on ethnographic research conducted between 2006 and 2010, this chapter presents a view from within a large-scale program that sought to manage local HIV responses and govern the participation of communities most highly affected by the HIV epidemic. Various business science logics and techniques—emanating from the large-scale, multi-state HIV program known as Avahan, funded by the Bill & Melinda Gates Foundation—gave rise to a culture of enumeration. The intervention did not merely act upon the intentionalities and social practises of people but it actually produced specific dimensions of sociality—subjectivities; social connections, affinities and tensions; organizational allegiances and oppositions; and cultural politics. Grafted onto epidemiological techniques of surveillance, Avahan's managerial hierarchy for governing the HIV response set in motion an enumerative regime that profoundly influenced local fields of possibility for community action. However, highly marginalized communities reworked these specialized knowledges regimes, putting them to practical use in meeting financial interests as well as concerns for health protection. At the same time, unintended negative consequences ensued when Avahan's modernizing discourses of individual empowerment ironically fractured the very networks of solidarity the program attempted to build for HIV prevention.

Keywords Mapping • Key populations • HIV prevention • Standards • Men who have sex with men

This chapter changes setting, to South India, but engages with a range of not unrelated notions of how community activism may transform itself as it becomes entangled in forms of science. The analytic perspective offered in this chapter, however, differs from the previous ones. Here my analysis presents a view from within a large-scale program that sought to manage local HIV responses and govern the participation of communities most highly affected by the HIV epidemic. Based on in-depth ethnographic research conducted between 2006 and 2010 in four districts of Karnataka, I learned how various business science logics and techniques—emanating from the large-scale, multi-state HIV program known as Avahan, funded by the Bill & Melinda Gates Foundation—gave rise to what Philip Setel has referred to

R. Lorway, *AIDS Activism, Science and Community Across Three Continents*,
Social Aspects of HIV 1, DOI 10.1007/978-3-319-42199-5_3

as "cultures of measurement."[1] By this I mean that the intervention did not merely act upon the intentionalities and social practises of people but it actually *produced* specific dimensions of sociality—subjectivities; social connections, affinities and tensions; organizational allegiances and oppositions, and cultural politics. At the same time new activist stirrings and networks of community solidarity emerged under the conditions of this expert-driven intervention.

The social transformations wrought by Avahan marked a departure from the sexual minority rights empowerment discourses that had previously inspired community collectives in India to respond to the HIV epidemic in the 1990s (Kavi 2007, Cohen 2005, Boyce 2007). Grafted onto epidemiological techniques of surveillance, Avahan's managerial hierarchy for governing the HIV response set in motion an enumerative regime that profoundly influenced local fields of possibility for community action. To begin to understand the forms of sociality and community politics ushered in by Avahan's intervention regime, and to properly locate the research I want to describe, this chapter outlines the architecture of the larger intervention and discusses how business logics combined with epidemiology to produce a surgically precise geography of intervention. I then show how social movement actors engaged with and unsettled Avahan's geography of intervention, investing in it to realize their own interests that well exceeded the expectations of those who designed and managed the large-scale program. As these highly marginalized communities become drawn in the project of governing access to sexual health services, their daily lived experiences reworked these specialized knowledges regimes, putting them to practical use in meeting financial interests as well as concerns for health protection. At the same time, unintended negative consequences ensued when Avahan's modernizing discourses of individual empowerment ironically fractured the very networks of solidarity the program attempted to build for HIV prevention.

3.1 The Architecture of a Business Model

Between 2003 and 2010, Avahan directed its financial management and clinical infrastructure to focus on the "most at risk populations" (sex workers, hijras,[2] men who have sex with men, people injecting drugs and male migrants) in the Indian states where the HIV epidemic was most pronounced, based on antenatal statistics and the epidemiological grand narrative of a "core-group" or "concentrated epidemic" (Fig. 3.1). Although the program originally intended to set up clinical services to detect and treat STIs and HIV among female sex workers, when men who

[1] Setel's notion is closely tied to the kinds of "audit cultures" discussed by Strathern (2000), where accountability practices are predicated on notions of efficiency and ethics.

[2] I sometimes refer to hijras as transgender males because many hijras today see themselves as distinct from men or women; a distinction that is reinforced by relatively newer state government regulations that allow hijras to claim a separate identity on voter and ration identification cards as "transgender."

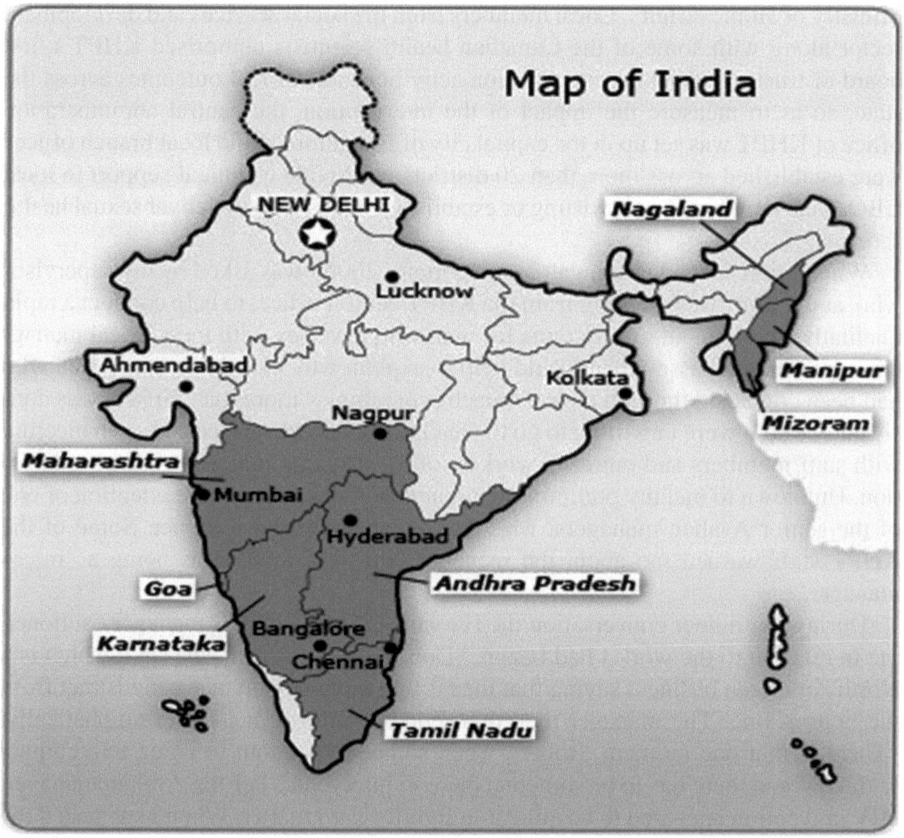

Fig. 3.1 Map of India's "High HIV Prevalence States": image created by AVERT

have sex with men and hijras began to present at these same clinics with a high disease prevalence (Go et al. 2004), the intervention specialists quickly realized that these groups also shouldered the burden of the HIV epidemic and thus needed to become a focus of the intervention.

According to literature made publically available by Avahan to promote its own accomplishments, this lavishly-funded program cost more than 330 $US million, and offered specialized services to more than 280,000 "most at risk populations" and approximately five million "men at risk," which included migrants across the high HIV prevalence states (Gates Foundation 2009). Avahan reported having partnered with 134 district-level NGOs and operated in 82 districts and 605 towns populated with approximately 200 million people. Directors of the program also formed close partnerships with the central government body in Delhi called the National AIDS Control Organization (NACO), and more than 20 organizations around the world, including academic institutions and nine international NGOs.

Public health scientists from the University of Manitoba, where I began my postdoctoral studies, formed one of these international NGOs, called Karnataka Health Promotion Trust (KHPT), which officially registered in 2003 with the Indian

Ministry of Home Affairs. Local members from the social services and development sector along with some of the Canadian health scientists comprised KHPT's first board of trustees. Tracking intervention activities and clinical outcomes across the state, so as to measure the impact of the intervention, the central administration office of KHPT was set up in the capital city of Bangalore while local branch offices were established across more than 20 districts to provide technical support to local CBOs that were either pre-existing or established in an effort to deliver sexual health services.

When I first arrived in Bangalore in February 2006 I was asked by my supervisor who, at the time, was working from the KHPT central office, to help conduct a rapid qualitative assessment of programs for men who have sex with men. Local managers hoped that the assessment could help to explain why exactly so many men who had been contacted through their outreach programs—"more than 50 %" I was consistently told—were unwilling to go to the clinic to access services. I began meeting with staff members and outreach workers of local sexual minority rights organization. Unknown to me, my preliminary research activities caught the attention of one of the senior Avahan managers, who then requested to have dinner. Some of the KHPT staff warned me about the manager who was reputed as being a "micro manager."

During our dinner conversation the Harvard-trained business manager cautioned me in relation to the work I had begun, "Don't boil the ocean" she said, which is a North American business saying that means that too much nuance can distract from the bottom line. The manager then proceeded to inform me, rather emphatically, "There is that one moment, Robert, when someone is about to come into contact with HIV and there has to be someone there to intervene." For the Avahan manager, HIV prevention appeared to be quite a straightforward matter. When I suggested the possibility that people may move in and out of various contexts of risk over the course of their life, the manager appeared irritated with my response and our meeting came to a rather abrupt end.

The injection of such private sector thinking into economic and health development is by no means new. Avahan continued the work of previous large U.S.-based philanthropic organizations, such as the Rockefeller and Ford Foundations, which infused their pioneering development work with free market ideologies, setting the stage for the more recent philanthropic work of Bill Clinton and George Soros. However, Avahan can be distinguished from previous generations of charitable aid to health and development in three ways: (1) the massive scaling up of funding to global health, following the donation of Warren Buffet's fortune to the Gates Foundation (McCoy et al. 2009; Ravishankar et al. 2009; Rogers 2011); (2) the intensified emphasis placed upon measuring and tracking of the donor's investment in economic and health development through ongoing mandatory reporting, enumerative procedures and the employment of business metrics, which define progress and performance of projects in quantitatively measurable terms (Bosworth 2011; Holmes 2015), and (3) the "augmented pattern of interaction between the donor (or 'investor') and the recipient (or 'investee')...in which investors facilitate skill and technical resource transfer, sustained relationship building and organizational support" (Moran 2009b:7). In the case of Avahan, this has meant that the Gates Foundation has not only provided ongoing financial support to India's HIV prevention programs but business personnel were also directly involved in its everyday management to closely track the progress of the foundation's investment.

The merger of the world of managerial science with public health under Avahan is reflected in the particular business logics employed by managers involved in governing the intervention. In a published interview, an Avahan program officer, Aparajita Ramakrishnan, explicitly draws an analogy between optimal health service coverage and the running of a successful business. She explains:

> Large businesses do not just implement in one little place, otherwise they don't make enough money. Similarly, with impact [of HIV prevention programs], I think you want to have a greater span. One of the ways to achieve this is…to be able to build an implementation pyramid. In other words, to be able to deliver services simultaneously across large geographies and across many populations. Then, some of the questions you can ask are: How do you manage the supply side to ensure that the product's sales force, in this case peer educators, are in the right place at the right time? Are they doing the right things? Is their job performance being measured? Do they have accountability? (Asthana 2008)

The role of market-oriented logics in Avahan's approach to health services delivery was also explicitly articulated by the Avahan director, Ashok Alexander, who stepped into his leadership role from the world of finance, as the former Director of McKinsey & Company, a prestigious management consulting firm. With close to 100 global offices, this company advises many of the world's most influential businesses and institutions. Along with Ramakrishnan, who also previously worked at McKinsey & Company, Alexander published "Avahan's Business Model" in the *Harvard International Review* in 2006. In general, the business model emphasizes entrepreneurialism, flexibility, technological innovation, and modern management practises, while trying to weave them together with public health principles. Also worthy of note, at the top of the model presented in the article is the phrase "the community"—which occupies a pivotal place in Avahan's intervention work. In fact, according to the literature that Avahan posted on their website, community participation is reiterated as the cornerstone of their program. Here is a short excerpt in which they cast "the community" as "the customer base."

> A business listens to its consumer. The community of sex workers is Avahan's respected consumer, and Avahan asks the community to define its needs. Avahan involves community members in program design and service delivery. (Ramakrishnan and Alexander 2006:60)

The emphasis placed on "community" in the Avahan business model can be traced to the ideas advanced by management theorist, C.K. Prahalad, in *The Fortune at the Bottom of the Pyramid: Eradicating Poverty through Profits* (2006) (also see Hammond et al. 2007). The "bottom" or "base of the pyramid" (BOP) theory, although contentious in scholarly arenas (see for example Karnani 2007), has served as a key guiding text in a new form of philanthropy termed "philanthrocapitalism" (Bishop and Green 2010)—a transformation in the history of organized "giving" that combines conventional approaches to charity with market logics and principles of investment arising out of venture capitalism.[3] According to the BOP theory, there are unmapped markets ("a fortune") that lie at the base of the social economic pyramid of the world's poor who make, on average, less than 2$ a day. According to this theory, this majority must not be considered merely as "poor victims". Rather, they must be viewed as "resilient and creative entrepreneurs," and as "value-demanding consumers." By supplying them with goods that they can buy and sell, the logic holds, they will not only be lifted out of poverty but will be, inevitably, socially and politically transformed. Thus, Avahan managers such as Ramakrishnan insist that "the reframing of development as enterprise, or targeting the poor as consumers, can contribute 'lasting solutions' that cannot be provided by traditional charitable relief" (Moran 2009a, b). For this reason, Avahan's vision of "success," in terms of sustainability, has come to hinge upon the participation of sex workers and sexual minorities, as Ramakrishnan explains:

> It's similar to any business model that you can find in the private sector, where there's a focus on the customer as the beneficiary of the services being sold – or delivered in the case of health. In the private sector that's buying toothpaste; in the public sector it might be the impact in terms of lives saved. In the context of HIV prevention in India, the recipients of prevention services (sex workers, men who have sex with men, injecting drug users) need to be part of the delivery, as peer workers (a 'sales force') and be leaders of community-based organizations delivering the interventions. So the question is 'Are you measuring everything you do, which is a very critical piece of any good business?'

Here impoverished sex workers are viewed as an untapped marketing resource or "sales force." By sales force Ramakrishnan means that the participation of sex workers in the intervention is expected to generate demand for health services—liberating a market force that will sustain the delivery of HIV prevention to highly stigmatized populations.

The community mobilization techniques devised by Avahan, which follow the business logics described by Ramakrishnan and Alexander above, have certainly proved effective for increasing the access of highly stigmatized communities to health services, at a grand scale. Moreover, it is important to note that the employment of this model has also yielded some striking results with respect to the reduction of curable STIs and HIV prevalence.[4] Yet how deeply do such approaches actually dig into the roots of social change to bring about the kind of lasting structural transformations needed to mitigate the social vulnerability of groups most at risk of HIV infection (also see Edwards 2009)? Arguably such logics fail to take critical stock of how the workings of capitalist forces actually rely upon and intensify

[3] "Philanthrocapitalism" was coined by Matthew Bishop and Michael Green. Mathew Bishop is the US business editor and New York Bureau Chief of The Economist. Michael Green is a London-based economist who has worked in aid and development for almost 20 years. He was a senior official in the British Government where he worked on international finance, managed UK aid to Russia and Ukraine, served three Secretaries of State as head of the communications department at the Department for International Development, and oversaw £100 million annual funding to non-profit organizations. Together they wrote "Philanthrocapitalism: How giving can save the world."

[4] See for example, the journal AIDS, December 2008, Volume 22, Supplement 5, 2008.

the production of social and political inequalities (and do so along the intersecting lines of gender, sexuality, race/ethnicity, caste, and so on).

3.2 Encountering the Geography of Intervention

The day after I first arrived in India, I was taken to the office of KHPT in Bangalore, the interior of which resembled an arrangement that one might expect to find in the private sector, with rows upon rows of uniform work stations separated by blue dividers. After being seated at one of the work stations assigned to visiting guests, and while I began opening up my laptop, a man with a wide, friendly smile walked towards my station to greet me, introducing himself as a demographer working on the monitoring and evaluation systems. He mentioned that he was currently engaged in a special behavioural study that was trying to capture how frequently "FSWs were having sex per week." Hiding some discomfort, I wondered to myself how having such information would actually help these women.

When I posed questions to the demographer about how the intervention was handling some of the social dimensions surrounding the HIV vulnerability of sex workers, he kindly printed off a set of indicators, some of which are depicted in Fig. 3.2. Learning that I was a social scientist, he was excited to tell me that they had recently included a number of new "structural indicators" related to violence committed by police and others who he referred to as "power structures"—that is, lovers, pimps, brokers, lodge owners, and *gharwalis* [madams]. The indicators were also utilized to enumerate the efforts made to mitigate violence and discrimination through what the demographer called "sensitization sessions" with police departments and district-level health officials. These were even designed to count the number of "key population" members (sex workers, men who have sex with men, and hijras) who received human rights and legal empowerment training. I found the number and breadth of the 66 indicators—ranging from "# of condoms distributed" to "# of people presenting with STI symptoms" to "# of incidents of violence reported", and so on—to be quite astonishing. I asked the demographer how they were able to gather all this information together and he explained that it came from the clinical records, the program data such as attendance sheets at trainings, and the daily tracking sheets used by the community mobilizers (see Fig. 3.3).

With respect to men who have sex with men and hijras, the community mobilizers in Bangalore were recruited from the large sexual minority rights organization known as Sangama, an entity that received some of its core funding from the Dutch humanitarian organization known as HIVOS, and thus emphasized human rights, anti-discrimination and legal protection issues in the organization's mandate. But as funding for sexual minority rights work began to dwindle, receiving funding from Avahan via KHPT became crucial for keeping the organization afloat.

Tracking sheets filled out on a daily basis by community mobilizers were an important part of outreach work used to measure some of the indicators around

Sl No	Indicator	Definition
1	Number of cities/towns covered	Total number of cities/towns that are covered by the program in the district. This number should not usually vary from month to month. However, if the program is expanded to newer cities/towns OR the program from a particular city/town is withdrawn in a particular month, add a note explaining why this number has changed from the previous month.
2	Number of villages covered	Total number of villages that are covered by the program in the district. This number should not usually vary from month to month. However, if the program is expanded to newer villages OR the program from a particular village is withdrawn in a particular month, add a note explaining why this number has changed from the previous month.
3	Number of sex work sites covered	Total number of sex work sites in both the urban and rural areas of the district that are covered by the program in the district. This number usually corresponds to the final list of sex work sites after validation and hence should not usually vary from month to month. However, if the program is expanded to newly identified sites within the cities/towns/villages covered, add a note explaining why this number has changed from the previous month. A sex work site is defined as a distinct area within the city/town/village where project outreach activity is planned. The site can be a public place, a lodge, a brothel, a dabha, or a home. In case of fixed places of sex work (such as the lodge, brothel, dabha or home), the site is the place of sex work.
4	Number of drop-in centers	Total number of drop-in centers in the district that are operational during the reporting month. A drop-in center is a definite venue, either within the NGO office or outside, provided for sex workers to meet. These centers may also provide other services to the sex workers. Count even if the drop-in centers that is part of the NGO office. This number usually should not vary usually from month to month, unless new drop-in centers are opened up or the earlier ones are not operational. In any case, provide a note explaining the difference, if this number varies from the previous month.

Sl No	Indicator	Definition
37	Number of sex workers who were diagnosed with anal ulcer	From among all the sex workers – new or repeat – who visited the clinic – program clinic, referral clinic or outreach clinic – during the reporting month, include only those who were diagnosed with anal ulcer. Count the number of individuals and not the number of visits. If a sex worker has visited the clinic twice during the reporting month, and on both the visits she/he was diagnosed with anal ulcer, count her/him only once. If the sex worker has visited the clinic twice during the reporting month, and on any one occasion she/he was diagnosed with anal ulcer, count her/him for this indicator.
38	Number of sex workers who were diagnosed with oral STI lesion	From among all the sex workers – new or repeat – who visited the clinic – program clinic, referral clinic or outreach clinic – during the reporting month, include only those who were diagnosed with oral STI lesion. Count the number of individuals and not the number of visits. If a sex worker has visited the clinic twice during the reporting month, and on both the visits she/he was diagnosed with oral STI lesion, count her/him only once. If the sex worker has visited the clinic twice during the reporting month, and on any one occasion she/he was diagnosed with oral STI lesion, count her/him for this indicator.
39	Number of sex workers receiving asymptomatic treatment[1] (first time only)	The number of sex workers that have received (either at the project clinic or the referral clinic or outreach clinic) asymptomatic treatment for Chlamydia and Gonorrhea for the first time in the reporting month. Individuals that are ongoing beneficiaries of asymptomatic treatment should not be included in this indicator.
40	Total instances of Asymptomatic treatment given	The number of times Asymptomatic treatment for Gonorrhea and Chlamydia was given in the reporting period. Includes those individuals that are ongoing or first time beneficiaries of asymptomatic treatment.
41	Number of sex workers treated with a Red pack	Count the number of sex workers who were treated with a Red pack during the reporting month. This is number of sex workers treated and not number of packs given.
42	Number of sex workers treated with a White pack	Count the number of sex workers who were treated with a White pack during the reporting month. This is number of sex workers treated and not number of packs given.
43	Number of sex workers whose partners are treated with a Blue pack[2]	Count the number of sex workers whose partners were treated with a Blue pack during the reporting month. This is number of sex workers treated and not number of packs given.
44	Number of sex workers treated with a Green pack	Count the number of sex workers who were treated with a Green pack during the reporting month. This is number of sex workers treated and not number of packs given.

Fig. 3.2 Sample of indicators used to measure program impact

Sl No	Indicator	Definition
48	Number of reported cases of Police violence: CUMULATIVE	Total number of police violence occurred so far in the project. This is actually the sum of all the episodes of police violence occurred during the periods prior to the current reporting month. Do not add the number of police violence occurred during the current reporting month.
49	Number of reported cases of violence by other power structures: NEW	Include only the new cases of violence by other power structures[3] occurred during the current reporting month.
50	Number of reported cases of violence by other power structures: CUMULATIVE	Total number of violence by other power structures occurred so far in the project. This is actually the sum of all the episodes of violence by other power structures occurred during the periods prior to the current reporting month. Do not add the number of violence by other power structures occurred during the current reporting month.
51	Number of reported cases of police violence redressed through meetings: NEW	Include only the new cases of police violence redressed through meetings during the current reporting month.
52	Number of reported cases of police violence redressed through meetings: CUMULATIVE	Total number of police violence redressed through meetings so far in the project. This is actually the sum of all the episodes of police violence redressed through meetings during the periods prior to the reporting month. Do not add the number of police violence redressed through meetings during the current reporting month.
53	Number of reported cases of police violence redressed through contests: NEW	Include only the new cases of police violence redressed through contests[4] during the current reporting month.

Fig. 3.2 (continued)

condom distribution and program attendance. I was somewhat troubled by the role that the daily tracking sheets were playing in community mobilization efforts. Back in Canada, I too had once visited "hotspots" like local clubs and connected with people in my social network to link them to the STI/HIV clinical services located at the AIDS Coalition of Nova Scotia. But how would the relations of trust I held with peers been affected if I were eliciting and recording such detailed information—would it not have formalized my interactions with my peers and diminish the rapport needed to connect them to community-run health services? From a theoretical perspective, I also wondered if this enumerative regime, more broadly, created a disciplining effect, in the sense that French thinker Michel Foucault articulated in *Discipline and Punish* (1977), as people were subjected to information collection itineraries? As men who have sex with men, hijras and sex workers became embroiled in daily record keeping, what was the effect on the collective political agency of the local CBOs, I wondered?

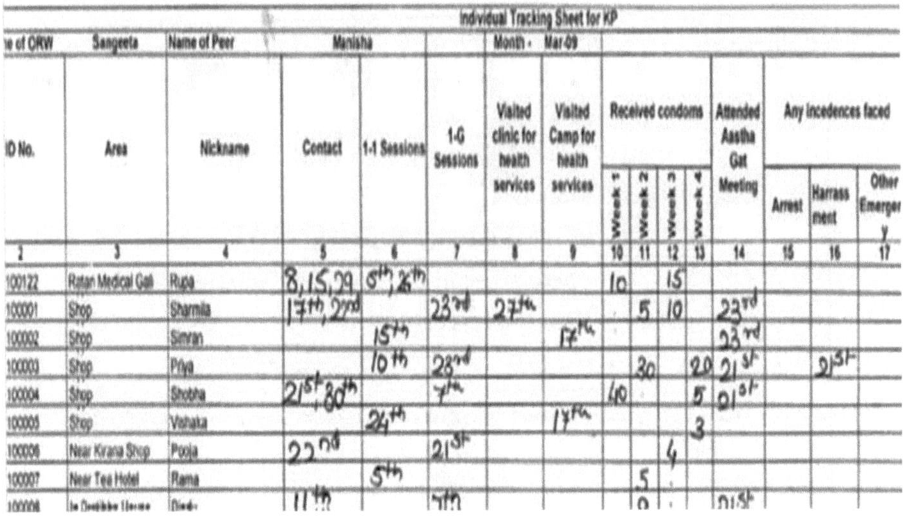

Individual Tracking Sheet for KP

...e of ORW	Sangeeta	Name of Peer	Manisha			Month - Mar-09										
ID No.	Area	Nickname	Contact	1-1 Sessions	1-G Sessions	Visited clinic for health services	Visited Camp for health services	Received condoms				Attended Aastha Gat Meeting	Any incedences faced		
								Week 1	Week 2	Week 3	Week 4		Arrest	Harrassment	Other Emergency
2	3	4	5	6	7	8	9	10	11	12	13	14	15	16	17
100122	Ratan Medical Gali	Rupa	8,15,29	6th, 26th				10		15					
100001	Shop	Sharmila	17th, 22nd		23rd	27th			5	10		23rd			
100002	Shop	Simran		15th			17th					23rd			
100003	Shop	Priya		10th	28th				30		20	21st		21st	
100004	Shop	Shobha	21st, 30th		7th			40			5	01st			
100005	Shop	Vishaka		24th			17th				3				
100006	Near Kirana Shop	Pooja	22nd		21st					4					
100007	Near Tea Hotel	Rama		5th					5						
100008	[illegible]	[illegible]	11th		7th				0			21st			

Fig. 3.3 Sample daily tracking form used by community mobilizers

Later that afternoon, I was invited to join one of the health promotion managers at KHPT, who took me into a small back office and started showing me a sexual typology diagram (see Fig. 3.4). He began by explaining the great lengths his working group made in constructing the following sexual typology:

Included in the diagram were a set of meeting notes that attempted to explain the terminologies. Here is an excerpt from the notes.

Working Group Meeting Notes

Western Separate Continuum: Theorists have challenged the binary system of gender and sex by arguing these identities exist on a continuum with the male and female as polar opposites and cross-, inter- and trans-gender (to denote the gradations of how individuals define their gender identity in contrast to their biological sex) in the middle. The continual but separate definitions of gender, sex, and sexuality imply that many different combinations of identities and orientations are possible.

Indian Fused Continuum: Gender, sex, and sexual identities and orientations exist continually, but represent themselves in a fused continuum with four main groups based on the combination of gender, sex and sexual identities with four main groups based on a combination of gender, sex and sexual identities and orientations.

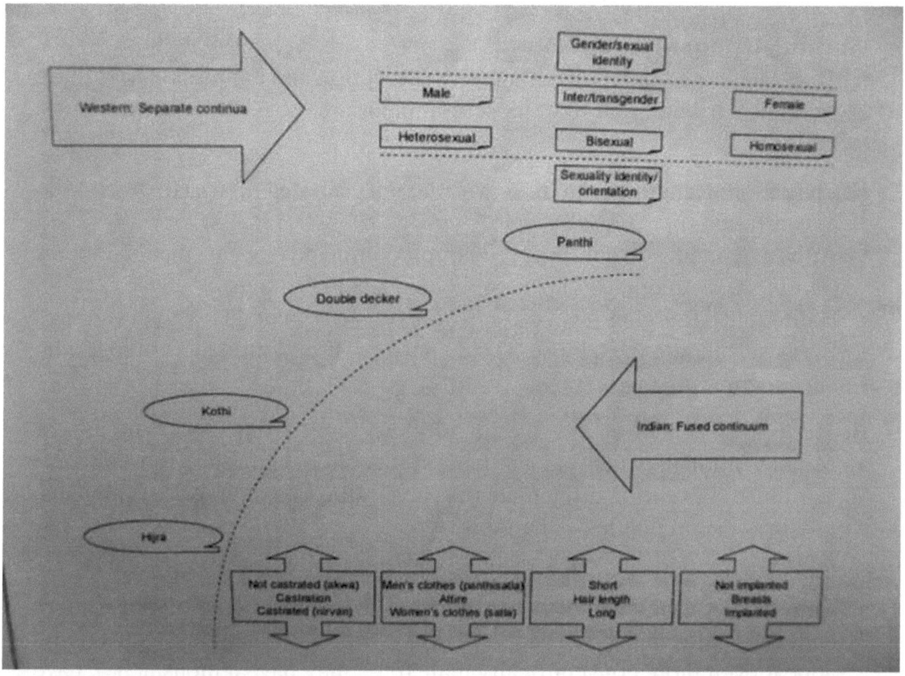

Fig. 3.4 Sexual typologies

In referring to "western sexualities" (toward the top of the diagram), represented by the arrow pointing to the right, the meeting notes specify a particular continuum of sexual and gender identities. This text related to Western sexualities appeared to me as a rather intriguing mélange of Western sexology and queer theory, with Judith Butler's (1989) repudiation of the "heterosexual matrix"[5] somehow thrown into the mix. As a contrast, the "Indian fused continuum" of male gender-sexualities was placed below the depiction of Western genders and sexualities. Then the meeting notes continued with a delineation of the four male gender-sexual categories that index physique, comportment, attire as well as desire as defining attributes of sexuality and gender.

[5] The heterosexual matrix interrogate a series of ideal relations assumed to exist between anatomical sex, gender expression and erotic desire (see Butler 1989: 259).

Working Group Meeting Notes

<u>Hijras:</u> There are gradations of identity perception and expression according to several attribute, but the most common are physical characteristics, including:

- Castration: Ranging from those who are not castrated (*akwa*) to others who are castrated (*nirvan*)
- Attired: ranging from those who predominantly wear men's clothes (*Panthisatla*) to others who wear women's clothes *(satla)*
- Hair length: Ranging from those who have short to others who have long
- Breasts: Ranging from those who do not have breast implants to those who have them

Hence, hijras' gender and sexual identity can range from those who appear more conventionally male (akwa, panthisatla, short hair, etc.) to other who appear more conventionally female (nirvana, satla, long hair, breast implants, etc.). Hijras desire panthis as partners.

<u>Kothis:</u>

- Thin line of difference between hijras, especially those who appear more conventionally male, and kothis, but we can define kothis as those who appear even more conventionally male (e.g., may have a moustache), have more conventional feminine mannerisms as well as desire men and possibly women.
- Some kothis want to be considered as hijras but don't want to undergo castration or wear saris, etc., are identified as chelas, a perceived lower social designation than hijras.
- Include some English-speaking, Western oriented Indian gay men.

<u>Double Deckers</u>

- Emerged in the last 4–5 years
- Can define double deckers as those who appear more conventionally male as well as desire men and possibly women, like their kothis counterparts, but may have more conventionally masculine mannerisms.

<u>Panthis</u>

- Considered amongst themselves and by their sexual partners as "real men"
- Perceive and readily identify themselves as heterosexual despite having sex with hijras, kothis and double deckers.

Some of my first thoughts related to the comparison drawn between western sexualities, which were portrayed as being more flexible, with multiple possible "combinations," in comparison to the "fused" Indian identities. This certainly stood in contrary to the gender and sexuality studies literature, which emphasizes the fluidity of South Asian sexualities (see for example Boyce and Khanna 2011). I also noticed that the "Indian fused continuum" was constructed along a rather curious-looking, almost evolutionary-looking arc, with the "descent of man"—the most masculine identity—appearing as fixed at the apex of the trajectory.

But what I found most puzzling was the fact that the working group felt it necessary to generate such a detailed characterization. I probed more into the background of the production of the typology. The manager said that the small working group consisted of leaders from communities of men who have sex with men and hijras, a CBO director, a social worker, an Indian health scientist and an American public health graduate student. The intent behind trying to produce clear delineations between these sexual identities related to the idea that the different groups had their own distinctive risks: "It is important that we are *knowing* the community, that we are understanding their risks," I was told by the manager.

The intensive effort on the part of the working group to "make-up" sexualities into a typological ordering scheme, coincided with the particular business logic of "segmenting the market," so as to narrow the aperture of the intervention to focus on the most at risk groups. The invention of such typologies was also an important part of how the managers and health scientists based in Bangalore and Winnipeg attempted to recreate standards (Timmermans and Epstein 2010) across the many intervention sites. Sexual typologies indeed enabled them to link together a multitude of sites throughout Karnataka State—covering wide and diverse geographies and domains of human experience and subjectivity—so that they could work together in the aim of "scaling-up" health service delivery. Interestingly, this process of making standards was not orchestrated entirely by experts, as the working group membership reflected; it also relied on community participation and insight. My conversation with the manager ended with two final comments: first, he said that some "MSM" do not even know their "real identity"; and second he informed me that "we are now getting the transgenders a vocal coach so they can sound more like normal women with higher voices."

The KHPT manager then introduced me to a group of frontline staff and community outreach workers who were waiting in an adjoined meeting room to further my orientation to their intervention. The public health staff introduced themselves using their names and educational credentials while each community member rhymed off their name and sexual identity label. For instance, one sex worker rose and introduced himself by saying "I am Raju and I am a double-decker because I am sexually versatile"; another man announced, "I am Rakesh, and I am a kothi because I feel like a woman." This all seemed rather rehearsed.

The production and reproduction of these sexual categories is perhaps better understood when viewed within the historical context of "state, bilateral and NGO-funded efforts to constitute culturally appropriate AIDS prevention interventions for men who have sex" in the 1990s (Cohen 2005:270). Lawrence Cohen's (2005) essay entitled "the Kothi Wars: AIDS cosmopolitanism and the morality of classification" discusses the heated public debate that broke out between two sexual minority-rights NGO directors—the UK born Shivananda Khan and the Indian journalist based in Mumbai known as Ashok Row Kavi. The source of contention was around Khan's assertion that the kothi (feminine male)-panthi (masculine male) dyad was an indigenous form of India male-male sexuality. Ashok Row Kavi challenged this claim of authenticity, insisting that it represented Khan's neocolonial imposition of order upon India sexualities which were more ambiguous and fluid than his typological scheme would suggest. In Cohen's own research, the terms kothi and panthi were unheard of in the regions of North India where he conducted his fieldwork prior to these debates, suggesting that these identity labels were a more recent invention than Khan had imaged. More important than the authenticity of these categories, however, these debates and the development work of sexual minority rights organizations in the 1990s led to the proliferation of male-male gender-sexual typologies throughout India. Furthermore, public health interventions further reified these categories as they mobilized communities for health services uptake (Boyce 2007).

On the second day of my orientation, the KHPT manager insisted that I join a team of other prevention specialists for a "field visit" at a local park to view how they had "mobilized" the community. I moved about the popular "MSM cruising spot," as they called it, on a late Saturday afternoon with four other health promotion managers who began pointing at individuals and firing out identity labels: "that one there is an MSW [a male sex worker], and that one is a hijra, she is transgender. The one waiting by the Banion tree is a CSW, a commercial sex worker. The one walking like a woman is called a kothi. And over there, he is a puka panthi (client), a real macho man!" I felt like I was on safari. Then they said, "Here are two of our community guides. Let's stop and talk with them and they can tell us about their work today." We stopped the car to meet with a small group of outreach workers who told us about how many condoms they had given out and how many "contacts" they had reached for that day. They were most pleased because they had exceeded their daily target.

Once my orientation at KHPT was completed, I began the rapid qualitative assessment in Bangalore, first by visiting the large CBO, Sangama, to gain an overview of the key health services-related issues facing the sexual minority rights NGO. Two community workers greeted me at the reception and self-identified as community mobilizers working on KHPT programs. The first individual, Suma, was dressed in a colourful green and golden-yellow sari and introduced herself to me as a "nirvana hijra" and a "community mobilizer." Suma explained that she had recently moved up the guru-chela hierarchy of hijras in recognition of her work as a community mobilizer. She no longer engaged in sex work; now she was responsible for providing room, board, and safer sex resources to her *chelas* (hijra disciples) (Reddy 2010:161).

The other self-identified community mobilizer, Fatima, introduced herself, by referring to her identity as a Kothi. She was a few years younger than Suma and wore men's clothing. She told me that she had wanted to have the castration operation but her parents forbade the procedure. As Suma and I began talking, Fatima repeatedly exited the room and re-entered, each time looking increasingly more feminine: first with lipstick, then eye makeup and then finally appearing with long dangling earrings. Her gate and comportment displayed an exaggerated, almost parodic, femininity, unlike that of Suma.

Soon the two mobilizers whisked me away in an auto-rickshaw and took me to an "MSM clinic," as they called it, near a large cruising park. I was led up the stairs into a community drop in centre and was seated on a mat at the front of the room before an audience of more than 30 people. Apparently, I was the main guest. Two hijras rose, and despite emulating a convincing presentation of femininity, began to speak using very loud, forceful and deep masculine voices to call the meeting together. Indeed the hijras were commanding in tone. My thoughts drifted back to the earlier meeting I had with the KHPT manager who said that hijras needed "voice lessons" to sound like "normal women with high voices." When I was first introduced to the community members at the KHPT offices, the same hijras seemed quiet and subdued while those identifying as kothis and double-deckers seemed more confident and outspoken. By contrast in the Sangama offices it was clear that hijras ran the show.

All the members introduced themselves using a name and their sexual identity label, which very much reflected the typological scheme that the KHPT working group had constructed. Some, however, introduced themselves as gay or bisexual and a number identified as "MSM." Initially, I had the impression that the use of clinical term "MSM" and other sexual typologies for self-introductions on a public health program exemplified the medicalization of sexuality, whereby people merely submitted to the typological scheme that had been imposed upon them by the epidemiologists, clinicians, and managers, so that they could be governed for the purpose of HIV health services delivery. However, as time went by, I came to learn that these communities bore deep affective attachments to these terminologies.

During the meeting, I was invited to explain the purpose of the rapid assessment. Then the group chimed in about their challenges as community mobilizers in getting their contacts to actually come into the clinic to access services. During the question period, the group began asking me numerous questions about genders and sexualities in Canada. People seemed most curious about how "the hijras in Canada," as they put it, were able to access "female hormones."

Following our conversation, many of the attendees stayed back to meet with me and to discuss, without my prompting, their sexual life histories, offering intensely personal narratives of their struggles with discrimination and violence. What struck me, as I listened, was that the sexual identifications they employed in their stories were deeply meaningful to this group. They not only facilitated their access to much needed health services but also these labels linked them to broader political goals, to a sense of belonging in the community, and to a sense of entitlement to social justice.

Suma and Fatimah then took me to the nearby cruising park, as the evening approached. We went off the main roadway toward the path in the grass where I was introduced to a few hijras and a woman who I was told was an "FSW" (female sex worker). Together the group showed me a small area where the police often harassed them "even those of us who give out health information are treated badly." One individual stated that they were sometimes arrested just for carrying condoms, even though they had the community mobilizer identity cards administered by KHPT.

As the sun began to set, we returned to the main road and continued to walk the entire length of the park. Along the way, my guides continually pointed to members of their community "that one there, you can see she is satla kothi. You can tell by how she is moving her body", "Over there, those are DD's, they are just cruising for sex but they are not selling" and "Look at that hijra there, she is one of my chelas." It would seem that community members not only held mastery over this geography of intervention but their engagement in the intervention was crucial to its animation.

3.3 Mapping Key Populations

The geographic mapping of key populations—an enumerative technique that generates population estimates of people defined as being at high risk for HIV infection—guided the production of standardized information on sexual difference and health service delivery across the wide geography governed by Avahan. Ultimately, geographic mapping procedures yield a spatial-temporal blueprint for measuring the distribution of "hotspots" and the "most at risk people" in a given catchment according to specific times (Lorway and Khan 2014). Managers and health scientists invested considerable financial and technical resources in geographic mapping, and the process itself was highly involved (for example see Emmanuel et al. 2010).[6]

Included among the team of scientists, health officials, and NGO directors who execute this procedure are community members, who serve as the field enumerators. These enumerators characterized and identified the hotspots and linked them to the predefined sexual typologies using a short survey tool. Once the mapping data is collected, M&E teams generate subpopulation size estimates and ascertain the high and low traffic periods for each of the locations according to days of the week and times of the day.

As a data set, mapping findings may be useful for measuring and setting program coverage targets. Because the mapping procedure generates population size estimates per units of space (i.e., "hotspot"), this enables outreach teams to work with a denominator—which is the number of high risk people they would need to reach to have "program saturation" (100 % coverage, that is). The actual number of people reached—the numerator—set against the denominator, may then be used to calculate the proportion of people a program is missing per zone. Because the mapping data also enumerates the peak times when people frequent hotspots, program manager are able to identify "program coverage gaps" in quantitative temporal as well as spatial terms. For community mobilizers, this mapping of hotspots can also serve as a blueprint for where and when they should conduct their outreach work.

[6] I further discuss the methodological details pertaining to geographic mapping in relation to evidentiary sovereignty in Lorway (2016).

Mapping data is also highly prized by the program managers because it helps to show, on the basis of enumerated hotspots and population concentration, where resources should be allocated, and how prevention technologies like condoms should be distributed (Emmanuel et al. 2010). By offering the possibility of multiple layers of spatial and temporal randomization, mapping data also serves as a highly desirable sampling template. Every couple of years or so, the mapping data was updated and used for special integrated biological and behavioural assessments (known as the IBBA) to measure the impact of the intervention on the HIV and STI epidemics. Together, these biological, behavioural and program monitoring and surveillance data were fed periodically to the external monitoring and evaluation team of experts known as CHARME—led by Indian, Canadian, and UK scientists who were tasked with modelling impact in terms of services delivered and number of infections averted. But the significance I want to draw attention to here is how geographic mapping fostered a way whereby intervention managers and Indian and Canadian health scientists came to view communities as definable, calculable, and governable subpopulations. Mapping data also enabled them to visualize the discrete locations in which the HIV epidemic was imagined to reside (Legg 2008; Brown and Knopp 2010:39).

The articulation of mapping and the typologization of sexual difference permitted visitors to the program to regularly observe the intervention's performance. I frequently witnessed how visiting scientists, health officials, and potential funders were taken on "field visits" to meet with community outreach workers based at different locals. Some prior staging and prompting always took place before the arrival of the guests, so that community mobilizers could properly perform their duties to meet the approval of the visitors. These inspection tours, as my colleague Shamshad Khan and I refer to them, enabled people working on the Avahan program to demonstrate their skill in spatially managing sexual minorities and associated "sexual risks" (Lorway and Khan 2014). The manner in which the sexual life of community members is put on display not only creates the illusion of order and control, but for Avahan, these regular inspection tours also allowed for the workings of the intervention to be "seen" by local and foreign monitoring and evaluation (M&E) specialists as well as prospective funders. In fact, I have witnessed on occasion how such field visits impress visiting donors to such a degree that they become the "selling point" for them to "invest" in the intervention. Inspection tours, therefore, function to foster confidence in the Avahan brand.

3.4 Clinic Life

The way mapping and enumerative technologies carved up and ordered space, forms the basis on which program managers and sex workers alike govern community access to specialized health services. During a community research project I coordinated with CBOs led by male sex workers and men who have sex with men in three districts of Karnataka between 2007 and 2009 (see Lorway et al. 2011), the community research team conducted participant observation at various hotspots so as to qualitatively capture "risk" from an environmental perspective. Their field notes illustrate the way intervention technologies, prevention discourses, and biomedical treatments have come to mediate the social connections between people.

> [At the park]: "You had your PTA [presumptive therapy assessment]?" We exchanged pleasantries and then he said "Where is the satellite clinic where we two can get [STI treatments]?" So, we went to the clinic. [I said] "This person needs PTA, it is due." [The physician said] "Ok bring the register from that room, get the ID number for the both of them." So I went with the card to the doctor.
>
> After we took the PTA and came to the market, the two left by bus. It was calm, people traded and waited for the buses. There I met a few kothis. One told me "sister, give me a chocolate [condom], a panthi [client] is calling me." I told her to be careful and to go only with decent guys as there are more instances of bullying these days.

This excerpt offers a glimpse into a social world that co-evolves with epidemic prevention; new "heterogeneous associations" (Latour 2005:5) between sex workers, clinicians, prevention discourses, treatments and pathogens are made possible by the ordered way of seeing sexualities and risk in spatial terms, seamlessly interweaving erotic and clinic life. Through attention to space, sex workers render "risk" legible for health promotion strategies at the same time as forging and reaffirming solidarities between community members. In the next excerpt, the description composed by a community mobilizer shows how epidemiologically oriented categories for sexual difference ("key populations") circulate as they connect men to health services and to communities of me how have sex with men.

> [The traffic hub] is a place where traders, labourers, students, owners, and doctors will come, one after the other, and this is a place where KPs [key populations] and hijras roam about seeking relaxation. A new guy came, he seemed nice. I asked him why he came here daily. He told me that when he watches those people sitting in groups, he gets a kind of feeling. "What kind of feelings are those?" I asked him. He stuttered and, biting his tongue, joined his hands in a [feminine] way. I asked him "K.P. [key population]?" He asked me back 'what does K.P. mean? I told him that people of our locality call such people who bite their tongue and act this way as K.P. or chakka [effeminate man].
>
> Then he agreed quietly that he was also of that kind. Later I convinced him to come to the DIC [community drop-in centre] to access our clinic. The technique of locating members of risk groups in space ("people of our locality") and time ("I asked him why he came here daily"), utilizes epidemiological categories as a technology for making up "the" community for the aim of meeting program targets. The technical application of sexual typologies in daily outreach work also enables community leaders to realize and execute citizenship projects that aim to rescue fellow members from anticipated danger.
>
> We entered into the bus station. In the toilet we found a kothi, getting prepared for oral sex. We were concerned, if the police find her, she will be beaten and harassed severely. We were quite vocal about it, to make her understand. She realized that we were trying to help and said "Thank you." We came out to the bus stand with her and sat on the benches. We asked her if she uses condoms while having sex. Her answer was a blatant "No!" We suggested using flavoured condoms during sex. We also told her that we distribute flavoured condoms in our office and she can come and take some. She asked if she has to pay for them. We said "No" and provided her with details of our DIC and the clinic… She confirmed that she would go but asked if I had a flavoured condom… I had two and gave them to her. I told her categorically that she should use condoms during sex, otherwise there is a

> very high chance of her getting infected and infecting others. She thanked me for the advice and left. I prayed for her well-being and welfare.

Outreach workers are not only instrumental in guiding the passage between risk (hotspots) and safety (the clinic), but they also act upon the geography of risk with their health protective strategies, remaking it with the distribution of condoms, the dissemination of safety awareness messages, and through referrals to specialized clinics and drop-in centres.

At this point in the story, one may wonder if the "working together" of a plethora of quantitative indicators, sexual typologies, tracking forms, and geographic mapping techniques has not established a "republic of enumeration" that local communities come to *serve*. As I interacted with the various CBOs over an extended period of time, a more complicated picture emerged, one in which collective political discourses and practises entwine with Avahan's enumerative regime, remaking the intervention techniques to serve their own interests.

3.5 Grounded Epidemiologies

With the passage of time, I came to notice that the participation of male sex workers and men who have sex with men in evidence production activities had shaped a particular way of "seeing like an epidemiologist." That is, they came to view themselves, their identities, communities and political struggles within strongly epidemiological frames of reference, although their usage was often driven by different interests. The narratives produced from the various community research projects I helped to coordinate were often teeming with multiple, partial and often ambiguous forms of epidemiological and biomedical knowledge, not unlike the medical creole discussed in Chap. 2. For practical and political ends, sex workers' daily practises retranslated, reinterpreted and re-assembled scientific ideas into what I call grounded epidemiologies. Take for example the map below (Fig. 3.5) drawn by male and transgender sex workers during the planning phase of a multi-district community research project.

I asked the group to discuss the map they had drawn and the many arrows that pointed to various locations and movements and which appeared somewhat puzzling. What was striking about their response was how they had taken what appeared to be a rather busy and hectic looking map and rendered it legible, in the sense that James Scott (1998) has articulated—that is, by constructing standardized explanations pertaining to when clients and sex workers flowed between various 'hotspots' throughout the city and according to particular days and specific time intervals. More intriguing was how the group assessed fluctuating levels of sexual risk and financial opportunities in precise temporal and spatial terms. When asked how they came to think like this, they explained further that "TLC" (time location cluster) sampling and other mapping exercises had helped them to become more organized in how they would go about sex work as well as protect their health. Other groups

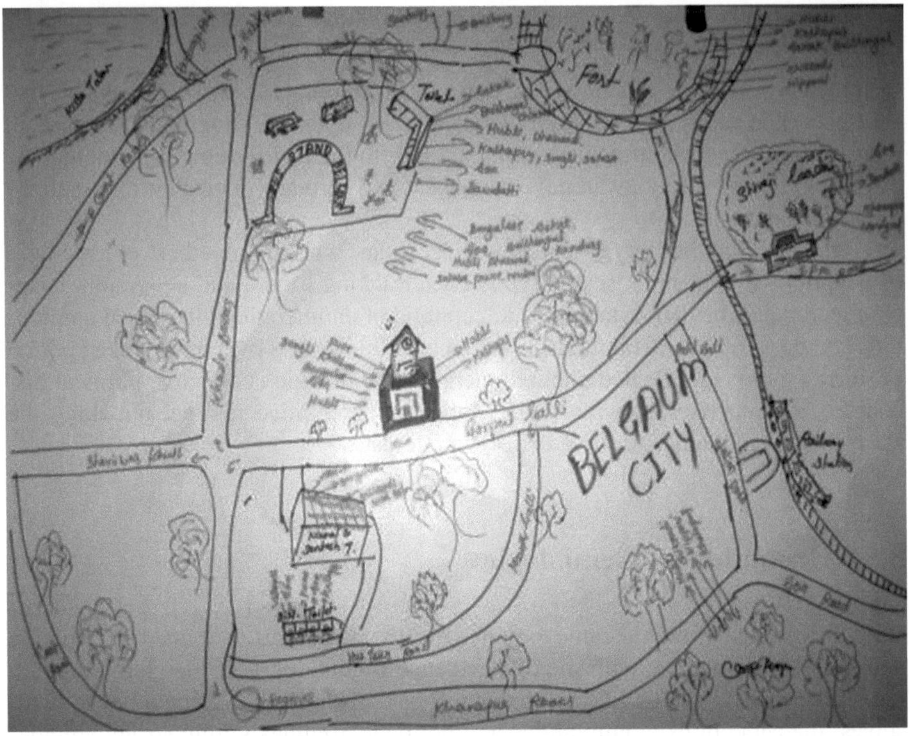

Fig. 3.5 Community map showing flow of clients across the city

joined in on the discussion and said that they often selected the districts, where they would go for sex work, according to the integrated biological and behavioural assessment (IBBA) findings. One male sex worker, for example, said "I hardly ever take clients around here, in Bellary, anymore because the HIV prevalence is just too high; it's 30 % now! I am only going to the lower HIV districts these days."

"Seeing like an epidemiologist" (similar to Biruk's term "seeing like a research project" (2012:351)) gestures to Scott's discussion of how modernist states deploy standardizing schemes to order and simplify society, rendering it manipulable for administrative purposes.[7] However, the re-working of surveillance knowledge through practises of self-governance, which confront the exigencies of sex work, suggests more than the extension of transnational power over local terrains of sexuality. The unexpected role of sex workers in the art of surveillance also speaks to the

[7] Here I also recognize that the work of governing the production of evidence, in the case of Avahan, unfolded "across a patchwork of transnationally networked bits" (Ferguson 2005:380, also see Biruk 2012:352).

tremendous successes that has been claimed under Avahan in terms of "HIV infections averted" (see for example, Banandur et al. 2013: 241).[8]

I insist that these grounded epidemiologies should not be regarded simply as lay versions that emerge in the leakage from the epidemiological "citadel" (Downey and Dumit 1997:6). Nor am I suggesting that these knowledges should be evaluated (either praised or dismissed) according to how closely they resemble supposedly legitimate scientific knowledge, practises or calculations, as some epidemiologists might insist. Instead these "sciences from below" (Harding 2008:5), although partial, ambiguous, and hybridized, point to vital sites in the co-creation of scientific knowledges where the everyday practises of sex workers "reassemble epidemiology" (Lorway and Khan 2014), continually altering the very objects that surveillance experts track over time. In this way, sex workers practises formed a crucial and creative part of the process of evidence production.

It was also not uncommon for the research participants to report that they had engaged in a number of harm reduction strategies through which they effectively reconstructed epidemiological and prevention knowledge. These strategies included partner selection (avoiding intoxicated clients who were likely to be unwilling to wear condoms); assessment of clients' STI symptoms (based on visual symptoms and genital odour); substitution of lower risk sexual practises (such as oral or thigh sex) for anal sex; and selection of districts to have sex where HIV prevalence was lower or where they felt their anonymity would be protected. Although IBBA monitoring and evaluation procedures captured aggregates of individual behavioural change as well as STI/HIV prevalence, this bio-behavioural assessment was unable to show the processes through which these changes actually occurred on the ground, i.e., through the ways sex workers act on their risk environments and re-employ scientific knowledges in the context of their daily lives, both adhering to and conflicting with accepted public health standards.

3.6 Zones of Exclusion

Avahan's geography of intervention hinged on the participation of sex workers and sexual minorities, with the logic that community mobilization would generate enough demand among their peers to sustain regular health services seeking after the Gates project ended. Ironically, the building of these solidarities and networks of community responsibility also produced particular "zones of exclusion" (Lorway and Khan 2014).

One Saturday afternoon in October 2007, Natesh and I walked together near the gate of Mysore Palace while talking to male sex workers. As it grew dark, Natesh

[8] Success was declared on the basis of estimates of the number of infections averted, as calculated by mathematical modellers (see for example: Banandur et al., J AIDS 2013: 87,000 infections averted over 5 years (2003–2008) in Karnataka; and Pickles et al., Lancet Global Health 2013: 606,000 infections averted over 10 years (2004–2013) in four southern Indian states).

commented on the various displays of masculinity playing out before our eyes. Young men in their late teens and early twenties streamed passed the male sex workers, inflating their chests and posturing themselves in a masculine way. "Those are the panthis [clients]" Natesh commented. For me, what appeared to distinguish them from the male sex workers, who were batting their eyes and swaying their hips, was the exaggerated performance of masculinity. I asked Natesh why the community outreach workers never tried to contact these panthis, as he called them. He quickly responded "they are not MSM". Looking puzzled I pressed further "but they are men who have sex with other men—right?" He then quickly and confidently responded "they are non-community—they just fuck and go". Noticing my confusion he continued "they are not taking [up] identities like we are; we call them panthis but they don't call themselves panthis or MSM—so they can't be mobilized. They are not like us. We are more feminine, you know, the kothis …."

There is, of course, a striking paradox here, when one considers the genealogy of the term, "MSM." As queer theorist and anthropologist Tom Boellstorff (2011: 291) explains "MSM was a scientific and bureaucratic coinage, created to signify behaviour without identity, as can be seen the originary form 'men who have sex with men but do not identify as gay.'" By contrast, for Natesh, like many other male sex workers I came to know, "MSM" was an important identification that granted feminine acting men access to specialized health resources, to social and political networks, while simultaneously eliding the health needs of more masculine acting men who did not take up sexual minority identities.

On another occasion, in May 2008, Natesh led me through a maze of hotspots one late afternoon, from railway stations to the city bus stand, from public parks to Hindu temples. Along the way, he pointed to an empty stadium where young men were smoking and congregating. He stated that the sex workers "there" were "bad and used drugs." Another outreach worker who had accompanied us that day added, "we must avoid them because they cannot be mobilized; they cannot be part of the community." A week later, another experienced outreach worker described a lodge that was popular with young male migrant labourers during the Diwali festival (where hijras frequently solicited them as clients) as "dirty and unclean—we don't mobilize in those places." Some male sex workers soliciting around the hotels where visiting tourist resided were referred to as "criminals" and were also avoided.

A couple of years later, I met up Natesh at the office. He seemed particularly agitated. "We need to meet in the field later today." After he helped some of the other sex workers fill out their contact sheets for the day, we left Ashodaya's office and headed toward the city bus stand, where we frequently met up with guys selling sex near the public toilets. In 2010, the bus stand was closed for renovation for almost the entire year, which really disturbed the sex work. Everyone at Ashodaya was excited that the newly renovated bus stand, which had undergone major "upgrading," was now open for business. As we approached the station, Natesh started pointing out various young men, who appear to resemble each other in the following ways: they wore tight red, green, or yellow t-shirts that displayed the Playboy logo, had earrings, and Nike sneakers. A few of them sported armband tattoos.

With the 2009 Delhi High Court ruling and de-criminalization of homosexuality, and the first ever gay pride parade held in Bangalore soon after, the visibility of small groups of cosmopolitan-looking young men began to mushroom throughout Mysore city. They often connected over Planet Romeo, a global gay dating website, before meeting up in public places. Once Natesh and I finally arrived at the bus-stand, he pointed out more groups of these young, trendy-looking guys. He exclaims "there are so many D.D.s now—calling themselves "Gs" [gays]. But they are not selling sex; they're doing it for pleasure. This is really bad for our business. They are having sex with our clients for free." Once his anger subsided, I asked Natesh and another guide who joined us if these D.D.s ever came to the office to access their sexual health resources. The other guide responds "We cannot mobilize them, because they are not wanting to be part of us, because we are sex workers, you know."

The theme of exclusion recurred during a community research training session in the northern Karnataka district of Belgaum. I asked the community researchers if there were any groups of sexual minorities who did not access their health services. They promptly mentioned the "jogappas" (male transgender devotees to the goddess Yellamma) who were characterized as "trouble makers and beggars; they are not part of our community." When I asked if they thought this group might be at a high risk for contracting HIV and STI, I was told that "they are not part of our community and they don't like our organization because we can't give them ration cards [to access social welfare resources]." Speaking with both the community leaders, who assisted with the IBBA recruitment, and members of the jogappa community, I learned that this group had not been recruited for the first round of the IBBA and initially were not mobilized to access services at their community DIC. In this way, the typological and spatial scheme employed by monitoring and evaluation specialists were retranslated by the community to mark the moral and political boundaries of community participation in ways that excluded a group of people from the intervention.[9]

These zones of exclusion reveal how male sex workers and sexual minorities utilize sexual typologies and Avahan's ordered outreach schemes in unexpected ways—to purify the boundaries of community participation. In other words, the way that intervention specialists typologized these communities to achieve the goal of "high risk group coverage" was reinterpreted by sex workers through the local moral demarcations of who resides in "the community" and who does not. But the continual re-drawing of these moral boundaries through exclusionary practises cannot be understood merely as the misapplication of the principles of epidemiology or management science employed in Avahan programs. Rather, these practises of exclusion expose something crucial about the very workings of the intervention's

[9] By including them in a couple of our studies in the region, the community research team soon learned that this group not only had very little knowledge of condoms and "safer sex" but they also shared many of the same clients as the male sex workers in Belgaum, which was revealed when we undertook a sexual network study (see Lorway et al. 2010). Thus the community eventually arrived at the conclusion that it was important to include Jogappas in their outreach work.

spatial-typological regime—namely, an appropriately mobilized community is one that can be presented in an orderly fashion. From the perspective of sex workers, certain types of people and places—cast as unmanageable or unruly outliers that threaten the "optics" of a successfully running project—become excluded from epidemic prevention.

3.7 Networks and Transactions

Kumar, a male sex worker, held out his mobile phone one day, showing a picture he had captured of Raju dressed in a sari. He teased him until Raju snapped back, angrily. I had worked closely with Raju over the years, teaching him how to create databases and how to enter and analyze data from various community research projects. In my early conversations with him, Raju had identified as "a DD" and a bisexual, but he claimed to feel more camaraderie with male sex workers, as he shared a similar social class background. As a community mobiliser, too, he would travel around with groups of male sex workers to check up on his contacts in the same places where he would cruise for sex. Although Raju met his sexual partners in the same hotspots that male sex workers found clients, and he hung around with a closely knit group of sex workers, he did not have sex for money. And while I had seen most of the male sex workers (at some point) wearing saris for self-pleasure, festivals, work, or for CBO "cultural events," Raju never wore satla [women's clothes]. So I was surprised to see the picture of him in a sari today.

Raju offered an explanation, saying that his family had fallen on hard times since his uncle, the bread winner of the family, had passed away. Now he was responsible for supporting his family. But he did not make enough money from his part-time CBO volunteer stipend. "Now, every Sunday I am having to do *basti* work," he explained. Basti work, as a term, means several things among kothis in Mysore who sell sex. Firstly, it refers to the act of blessing shops. A number of male sex workers in Mysore dress in saris and travel to Bangalore in the day to take donations for basti work, blessing shops in the city or seeking small donations from drivers in high density traffic areas. Some of them travel back in the evening to Mysore where they wear panthi satla (men's clothes) and sell sex at the bus-stand, the railway station or public parks. Basti work, however, was not only associated with blessing shops or begging but also the act of selling sex. Raju was referring to the lattermost meaning here.

Although Raju seemed upset about entering into regular sex work, he insisted he was also deeply grateful to the friendships he had made at the local CBO in Mysore, as he was able to quickly build up a clientele base to help support his family. His peers generously referred some of their clients to him. He hated wearing saris, he said, but he was able to make a lot of cash when he dressed like a woman. Raju expressed to me his concern over what he perceived as an elevated risk of infection for HIV and other STIs. "Now I am having to do a lot more anal sex because clients expect it. Before when I was doing it for pleasure, I was having mostly oral sex. It was much safer."

The primary aim of Avahan's community mobilization strategies has been to connect sex workers to health services and track progress in terms of program coverage. What I observed, however, was how these regimes of intervention were also implicated in the reconfiguration of the social and sexual networks of sex workers, creating increased financial opportunities. Overtime, groups of sex workers not only began to work together on community health and safety projects (i.e., STIs treatment, confronting police and goondas violence, and condom distribution, and so on; see, for example: Argento et al. 2011; Reza-Paul et al. 2012) but they cooperated in mobilizing finances. The very intervention techniques employed to enhance community participation were also used to mobilize flows and accumulations of capital, accumulations regulated by local hierarchies of respect, funnelled through social network channels. For instance, when male sex work community leaders went to local, national, and international conferences or training opportunities, they would often refer their clients to their trusted peers, who were usually more senior members within CBOs, so as not to lose this income source. When I asked a group of 20 or so male sex workers in Mysore why they shared clients, one man responded "We can make sure the clients are safe and using condoms, and it is also good for business. Clients want to try it with different sex workers, but this way we keep the business in our group."

3.8 The Phantom Phallus and the "High-Tech Hijra"

Hijras, referred to by some academics and rights activists as a "third sex," have occupied a socially accepted religious role since ancient times (Nanda 1990). Today they continue to perform and give blessings during weddings, births and earn a living through their *basti* work. Nevertheless, hijras have also become extremely socially marginalized, impoverished and, coupled with their regular practise of sex work, extremely vulnerable to HIV infection (Reddy 2005).

With the descent of HIV interventions upon the State of Karnataka, the notion of hijras as a culturally distinctive sex has begun to shift toward more Western biomedical definitions of transgender bodies. Historically, hijras have undergone castration by removing the external genitalia through a ritualized process that posed significant health risks, and which leaves only an opening for urination. Increasingly, hijras are now electing to take hormonal replacement, have breast implants and undergo partial or full vaginal reconstruction, depending on how much money they are able to save.

The fostering of new norms of health service seeking among gender nonconforming males has certainly increased their access to safer castration procedures. Medical professionals in more cosmopolitan cities like Bangalore provide castration surgeries and vaginal reconstruction on medical grounds to get around laws prohibiting castration. In smaller and less cosmopolitan cities, such as Bellary, some local doctors have also begun to perform these surgeries, as doctors can earn more than 300,000 rupees (roughly 7500USD) per operation. Thus a new and unexpected enterprise has arisen around the Avahan intervention. The increased access to biomedical technologies also holds serious implications for local community support networks.

Historically young aspiring hijras, or chelas, became part of hijra clans (a hierarchical social structure between gurus and chelas). Over an extended period of time, and through ritualistic social practises that established their membership within a particular clan, chelas eventually may elect to undergo traditional castration ceremonies. More recently, however, among some of the young men who actively participate in the intervention, I have witnessed the acceleration in the process of undergoing castration, made possible by medical operations. A few young men have expressed considerable regret after too hastily having made the choice to become castrated. For example, one young man I will call Renu, who is a leading community mobilizer for his CBO in Bellary went in one day, spoke to the doctor, booked his operation and then, only a few days later, received the castration surgery. His friends were deeply upset that he had the surgery without consulting with them to make sure that he was certain of his decision. And Renu, himself, was at a loss to explain how quickly it had all happened. On one occasion, Renu spoke with me about his amputated body and how he would wake up in the middle of the night, feel that his genitalia were still present and then realize, regretfully, what he had done.

The rather extreme example of Renu's "phantom phallus" is not intended to suggest that doctors are coercing young men to undergo these operations or that the larger intervention is somehow responsible for the tragedy experienced by individuals like Renu, per se. It does, however, vividly call attention to the increasing speed through which sexual minorities are being "made," as a set of intervention techniques smooth the social pathways to assuming sexual identifications. These are, in other words, inadvertent negative side effects of Avahan's intervention technologies that are tied to the ethics of expediency, the concomitant compression of time, and emerging desires to be counted among those who can take responsibility for epidemic prevention and saving lives. Through the enumeration of daily life, sociality and modes of being rapidly transformed in ways that neither afford individuals the time to adequately negotiate their place in the community nor to reflect upon the new meanings and values that were attaching themselves to ideas of selfhood. Such accidental amputations recall the ideas of social theorist Paul Virilio (1986) on the tyranny of speed and the effects of technology, whereby the creation of new technologies also engineers "the accident," the "negativity" that always plagues the progress of the technology.

The ironic individualizing effect of community mobilization was also exemplified in the emergence of a new identity, known locally as "the high-tech hijra". These hijras are called "high tech" because they connect with their clients through cell phones and do not distribute their earnings through the traditional guru-chela clan system. Local community members frequently criticized them as acting as though they are "above" ordinary hijras. One hijra explained to me that high tech hijras operated more like individuals while her friend continued by saying: "They have wealthy clients and some can even afford to have full vaginal and facial reconstruction."

The emergence of high tech hijras, particularly in Bangalore, can be linked to the unprecedented urbanization and economic transformation that has occurred in the region due to the boom in the information technology industry; there are more intense circulations of financial capital that can be captured through sex and basti work. However, these new identities are also ushered in through the networks of health promotion organizations working in association with Avahan. Various district-level program managers I have met have celebrated the success of their empowerment work with hijras and female sex workers by suggesting how they have come to start to resemble and even become indistinguishable from the more middle class female health promotion staff working with them. On one hand, the regular contact between middle class intervention managers and hijras and other sex workers has positively changed how many hijras come to see their relation to society—as being less marginal. However, within the context of the intervention the emergence of the "high tech hijras" as those who distances themselves from the previous guru-chelas clan system, both economically and socially, points to modernizing locations whereby community networks of solidarity—the very resources that intervention specialists seek to cultivate—are breaking apart.

References

Asthana, A. (2008). *Avahan India AIDS initiative: Interview with Aparajita Ramakrishnan*. http://www.globalhealthdelivery.org/blog/2008/08/avahanindia-aids-initiative-interview-with-aparajita-ramakrishnan/

Argento, E., Reza-Paul, S., Lorway, R., Jain, J., Bhagya, M., Fathima, M., Sreeram, S. V., Hafeezur, R. S., & O'Neil, J. (2011). Confronting structural violence in sex work: Lessons from a community-led HIV prevention project in Mysore, India. *AIDS Care, 23*(1), 69–74.

Banandur, P., Mahajan, U., Potty, R. S., Isac, S., Duchesne, T., Abdous, B., Ramesh, B. M., Moses, S., & Alary, M. (2013). Population-level impact of Avahan in Karnataka state, south India using multilevel statistical modelling techniques. *JAIDS Journal of Acquired Immune Deficiency Syndromes, 62*(2), 239–245.

Biruk, C. (2012). Seeing like a research project: Producing "high-quality data" in AIDS research in Malawi. *Medical Anthropology, 31*(4), 347–366.

Bishop, M., & Green, M. (2010). *Philanthrocapitalism: How giving can save the world*. New York: Bloomsbury Publishing.

Boellstorff, T. (2011). But do not identify as gay: A proleptic genealogy of the MSM category. *Cultural Anthropology, 26*(2), 287–312.

Bosworth, D. (2011). The cultural contradictions of philanthrocapitalism. *Society, 48*(5), 382–388.

Boyce, P. (2007). 'Conceiving kothis': Men who have sex with men in India and the cultural subject of HIV prevention. *Medical Anthropology, 26*(2), 175–203.

Boyce, P., & Khanna, A. (2011). Rights and representations: Querying the male-to-male sexual subject in India. *Culture, Health & Sexuality, 13*(1), 89–100.

Brown, M., & Knopp, L. (2010). Between anatamo-and bio-politics: Geographies of sexual health in wartime Seattle. *Political Geography, 29*(7), 392–403.

Butler, J. (1989). Gendering the body: Beauvoir's philosophical contribution. In *Women, knowledge, and reality: Explorations in feminist philosophy* (pp. 253–262). Boston: Unwin Hyman.

Cohen, L. (2005). The Kothi wars: AIDS cosmopolitanism and the morality of classification. In S. Pigg & V. Adams (Eds.), *Sex in development: Science, sexuality, and morality in global perspective*. Durham: Duke University Press.

Downey, G. L., & Dumit, J. (Eds.). (1997). *Cyborgs & citadels: Anthropological interventions in emerging sciences and technologies* (pp. 245–264). New Mexico: School of American Research Press.

Edwards, M. (2009). Gates, Google, and the ending of global poverty: philanthrocapitalism and international development. *The Brown Journal of World Affairs, 15*(2), 35–42.

Emmanuel, F., Blanchard, J., Zaheer, H. A., Reza, T., & Holte-McKenzie, M. (2010). The HIV/AIDS Surveillance Project mapping approach: An innovative approach for mapping and size estimation for groups at a higher risk of HIV in Pakistan. *AIDS, 24*, S77–S84.

Ferguson, J. (2005). Seeing like an oil company: space, security, and global capital in neoliberal Africa. *American Anthropologist, 107*(3), 377–382.

Gates Foundation. (2009). *Avahan AIDS Initiative Commitment Increased to $338 Million – Bill & Melinda Gates Foundation* (Press release July 2009). http://www.gatesfoundation.org/Media-Center/Press-Releases/2009/07/Avahan-AIDS-Initiative-Commitment-Increased-to-$338-Million.

Go, V. F., Srikrishnan, A. K., Sivaram, S., Murugavel, G. K., Galai, N., Johnson, S. C., Sripaipan, T., Solomon, S., & Celentano, D. D. (2004). High HIV prevalence and risk behaviors in men who have sex with men in Chennai, India. *JAIDS Journal of Acquired Immune Deficiency Syndromes, 35*(3), 314–319.

Hammond, A. L., Kramer, W. J., Katz, R. S., Tran, J. T., & Walker, C. (2007). *The next 4 billion: Market size and business strategy at the base of the pyramid*. Washington, DC: World Resources Institute International Finance Corporation.

Harding, S. (2008). *Sciences from below: Feminisms, postcolonialities, and modernities*. Durham: Duke University Press.

Holmes, G. (2015). Philanthrocapitalism, biodiversity conservation and development. In *New philanthropy and social justice: Debating the conceptual and policy discourse* (p. 81). Bristol: Policy Press.

Karnani, A. G. (2007). *Mirage at the bottom of the Pyramid* (SSRN working paper series). http://deepblue.lib.umich.edu/bitstream/handle/2027.42/57215/wp835?sequence=1.

Kavi, A. R. (2007). Kothis versus other MSM: Identity versus behaviour in the chicken and egg paradox. In *The phobic and the erotic: The politics of sexualities in contemporary India* (pp. 391–398). London: Seagull Books.

Latour, B. (2005). Reassembling the social-an introduction to actor-network-theory. In B. Latour (Ed.), *Reassembling the social-an introduction to actor-network-theory* (p. 316). Foreword by Bruno Latour. Oxford University Press, September 2005. ISBN-10: 0199256047. ISBN-13: 9780199256044, 1.

Legg, S. (2008). *Spaces of colonialism: Delhi's urban governmentalities*. New York: Wiley.

Lorway, R. (2016, January). *What's your denominator?: Standardizing HIV/AIDS service delivery in Kenya*. Paper presented at the "Making Standards" conference, Dalhousie Univeristy.

Lorway, R., & Khan, S. (2014). Reassembling epidemiology: Mapping, monitoring and making-up people in the context of HIV prevention in India. *Social Science & Medicine, 112*, 51–62.

Lorway, R., Shaw, S. Y., Hwang, S. D., Reza-Paul, S., Pasha, A., Wylie, J. L., Moses, S., & Blanchard, J. F. (2010). From individuals to complex systems: Exploring the sexual networks of men who have sex with men in three cities of Karnataka, India. *Sexually Transmitted Infections, 86*(Suppl 3), iii70–iii78.

Lorway, R., Hwang, S. D., Reza-Paul, S., Pasha, A., Rahman, S. H. U., Moses, S., & Blanchard, J. (2011). Sex in the city: Privacy-making practises, spatialized intimacies and the environmental risks of men-who-have-sex-with-men in South India. *Health & Place, 17*(5), 1090–1097.

McCoy, D., Chand, S., & Sridhar, D. (2009). Global health funding: How much, where it comes from and where it goes. *Health Policy and Planning, 24*(6), 407–417.

Moran, M. (2009a). Philanthropic foundations and global health partnership formation: The Rockefeller Foundation and IAVI. In S. MacLean, S. Brown, & P. Fourie (Eds.), *Health for some: The political economy of global health governance* (pp. 118–129). Basingstoke: Palgrave Macmillan.

Moran, M. (2009b). *New foundations, the new philanthropy and sectoral 'blending' in international development cooperation.* Paper presented to the Australasian Political Studies Association conference Macquarie University, Sydney, Australia, 7. Retrieved from http://researchbank.swinburne.edu.au/vital/access/manager/Repository/swin:20047.

Nanda, S. (1990). *Neither man nor woman: The hijras of India.* Belmont: Wadsworth Publishing Company.

Pickles, M., Boily, M.-C., Vickerman, P., Lowndes, C. M., Moses, S., Blanchard, J. F., Deering, K. N., et al. (2013). Assessment of the population-level effectiveness of the Avahan HIV-prevention programme in South India: A preplanned, causal-pathway-based modelling analysis. *The Lancet Global Health, 1*(5), e289–e299.

Prahalad, C. K. (2006). *The fortune at the bottom of the pyramid.* Upper Saddle River: Pearson Prentice Hall.

Ramakrishnan, A., & Alexander, A. (2006). Practicing theory: Management in HIV intervention. *Harvard International Review, 28*(2), 58.

Ravishankar, N., Gubbins, P., Cooley, R. J., Leach-Kemon, K., Michaud, C. M., Jamison, D. T., & Murray, C. J. (2009). Financing of global health: Tracking development assistance for health from 1990 to 2007. *The Lancet, 373*(9681), 2113–2124.

Reddy, G. (2005). Geographies of contagion: Hijras, Kothis, and the politics of sexual marginality in Hyderabad. *Anthropology & Medicine, 12*(3), 255–270.

Reddy, G. (2010). *With respect to sex: Negotiating Hijra identity in south India.* Chicago: University of Chicago Press.

Reza-Paul, S., Lorway, R., O'Brien, N., Lazarus, L., Jain, J., Bhagya, M., Mary, P. F., Venukumar, K. T., Raviprakash, K. N., Baer, J., & Steen, R. (2012). Sex worker-led structural interventions in India: A case study on addressing violence in HIV prevention through the AshodayaSamithi collective in Mysore. *The Indian Journal of Medical Research, 135*(1), 98.

Rogers, R. (2011). *Why philanthro-policymaking matters.* Society, *48*(5), 376–381.

Scott, J. C. (1998). *Seeing like a state: How certain schemes to improve the human condition have failed.* New Haven: Yale University Press.

Strathern, M. (2000). *Audit cultures: Anthropological studies in accountability, ethics, and the academy.* New York: Psychology Press.

Timmermans, S., & Epstein, S. (2010). A world of standards but not a standard world: Toward a sociology of standards and standardization*. *Annual Review of Sociology, 36*, 69–89.

Virilio, P. (1986). *Speed and politics: An essay on dromology* (M. Polizotti, Trans.). New York: Semiotext(e).

Chapter 4
Documenting Sovereignty

Abstract This chapter recounts the details of a participatory research project that took place in Mysore, southern Karnataka. Compellingly, a vital form of collective action grew that exceeded the initial project's goal of generating knowledge around the effects stigma on health services access. The sparking of a social justice collective occurred because the participants seized the project to realize their own visions of community health. The participatory process of generating forms of knowledge that resonated with and could be readily understood by peers created a space in which an emergent collective of male sex workers began to assert their own interpretations of sexual health needs and problems. Of course these alternative knowledges did not entirely depart from Avahan's technocratic rendition of community health—for in fact, the collective continued to draw upon the expert knowledges and enumerative techniques that governed the larger response in the region. Furthermore, this participatory project operated by setting up new relations of power and inequality even as it moved to undo prevailing ones. When Avahan transitioned all of its community-centred intervention programs in India to the public system between 2010 and 2013, community-centred interventions were placed under the jurisdiction of the central government body, the National AIDS Control Organization, which flowed funds to the State AIDS Control Societies. As community activists and health workers become mired in paperwork, the fate of "community innovation" promoted under Avahan is revealed.

Keywords Avahan • Documents • HIV prevention • Bureaucracy • India

Although the geography of intervention described in that previous chapter tended toward the taming of political dissidence via standardized "community mobilization" schemes designed to link sex workers to health services and to track health services delivery (Lorway 2013), it also generated friction at the moments when it collided against the interests of members of local social movements, thus sparking forms of resistance and unexpected consequences. Through the lens of participatory research projects conducted with communities of sexual minorities across four districts of Karnataka State, I came to witness how the intermingling and co-evolution of identity politics, health protection discourses, business interests, and intervention techniques dramatically shaped the contours of social movements, reconfiguring

R. Lorway, *AIDS Activism, Science and Community Across Three Continents*, Social Aspects of HIV 1, DOI 10.1007/978-3-319-42199-5_4

them around managerial and epidemiological scientific rationalities (see Lorway and Khan 2014).

In this chapter, I explore one particular participatory research project that took place in Mysore, southern Karnataka. Compellingly, a vital form of collective action grew that exceeded the initial project's goal of generating knowledge around the effects stigma on health services access (Lorway et al. 2014). The sparking of a social justice collective occurred not because of my own efforts or intentionality as a researcher; but because the participants seized the project to realize their own visions of community health. The participatory process of generating forms of knowledge that resonated with and could be readily understood by peers created a space in which an emergent collective of male sex workers began to assert their own interpretations of sexual health needs and problems. Of course these alternative knowledges did not entirely depart from Avahan's technocratic rendition of community health—for in fact, the collective continued to draw upon the expert knowledges and enumerative techniques that governed the larger response. Furthermore, this participatory project operated by setting up new relations of power and inequality even as it moved to undo prevailing ones.

Community-based participatory research has gained considerable acceptance in recent decades given its ability to address social inequities, improve health outcomes, and enhance community participation and ownership with respect to various health-related interventions (Cornwall and Jewkes 1995; Israel et al. 2005). However, it must also be recognized that cultivating "participation" may not be entirely a straightforward, "liberatory," or positive transformative process. The critical social science and health literature is awash with examples of the paradoxical effects of participatory health and development projects that seek to "empower" oppressed communities but which unwittingly constitute new forms of inequality by diffusing and more deeply embedding the regulatory power of public health authority within local contexts (Lupton 1995). Furthermore, community participation can be uneven, temporary, sporadic, and, in some instances, burdensome for the community that is expected to sustain its outcomes beyond project funding (Cornwall and Jewkes 1995).

Without ignoring the inevitability of unequal power relations with respect to the process I coordinated, it is important to also recognize how the community of male sex workers was able to reposition their interests in larger policy arenas that governed their role in the HIV response. By opening up a space for a ground of evidence that mattered to affected communities, these sex workers were able to confidently launch their own broader political agenda, beyond the boundaries of the research project and the larger Avahan program. Eventually the affective networks and informal interactions set in motion by the participatory project evolved into a more formalized social movement. Although "un-measurable" by Avahan success indicators, the considerable influence that the male sex worker activist group came to wield in local and state policy arenas nevertheless must be tied to Avahan, which lauded the role of community participation, and provided a steady stream of resources that supported such goals under the banner of "community mobilization" and innovation.

4.1 Participatory Research Beginnings

The auto-rickshaw sputters and grinds to a halt, giving off oily kerosene fumes. I haggle with the driver for a while, who tries to raise the price we had originally agreed upon. After finally giving up and paying what the driver demands, I exit and look around. I am surrounded by shops selling used car parts. Young men are repairing tires, and nimbly throwing them up onto enormous piles. I notice a small Hindu temple, wedged between one of the mechanic shops and a small tea stall cum restaurant. A roadside stand sells rice and sambar. The fragrant smell of spice draws a small crowd of men.

Finally noticing the entrance of the CBO, I walk up a narrow flight of concrete stairs, in a small three story building. The buzz of voices speaking in Kannada grows louder as I reach the top. Peering in, I see pairs of people busily talking over each other, sitting face-to-face across small desks, filling out spreadsheet after spreadsheet.

A young man looks up from his desk and rushes toward me with a big smile: "Welcome to Ashodaya Samithi. We're a sex worker CBO, run by sex workers, sir." He seems most proud of the organization.

The local director of the Avahan intervention, an Indian physician and public health specialist, also warmly greets me as she guides me toward the boardroom. On the way, she notices me watching the enthusiastic form filling. "Those are the community mobilizers. They are filling out their contact lists, so they can keep track of their daily targets."

I enter the boardroom where a young group of men are gathered—they seem particularly excited to begin their presentation. The local health promotion staff members, who manage the day to day running of the intervention, begin by introducing themselves. They state their first name and their academic credentials. They are mostly trained in social work. The group of young men who crowd around the opposite end of the long board table follow suit. But instead they introduce themselves with their name and a sexual identity label. One man, for instance, says with great pride: "I am Shiva (pseudonym) and I am CSW [commercial sex worker] for five years." The others used a variety of other labels as a way of introduction, such as MSM, kothi, DD, hijra, TG and MSW.

Later in the day I learn that Shiva holds a Master's degree in business. I ask him why he and the others introduced themselves using sexual identities labels. He responds sharply: "We are the key population members." In other words, these identities were, in some way, their credentials that helped to establish their legitimacy as the rightful participants and beneficiaries of the intervention.

To provide background for me to understand the intervention they were running, the group begins to discuss a modified version of what they called "capture–recapture." This technique, they explain, estimates the size of the community.

The director interjects. "This procedure originally comes from the biological sciences; it has been used to estimate fish population sizes. But together, with the community, we have adapted it by turning it into a lottery."

With the LCD projector now warmed up, the formal presentation begins. A Google map segment of the city centre is presented. Small stars mark the "hotspots," as they called them, to indicate the most vibrant places where people congregate for sex work, for cruising and for casual outdoor sex. These hotspots are further grouped on the map into zones—forming a sort of blueprint for daily outreach work. The male sex workers in the group expressed particular concern about their "program coverage" as "50 % of their MSM contacts" (a figure stated in a tone of certainty) refused to come to the clinic or attend other programs offered at their drop in centre.

Following the presentation, the group decides that I should be taken on a "field visit" to meet with their other outreach workers and members of the community who worked at the various hotspots. I visit the city bus stand, a public park, and then some busy street intersections where my guide, a male sex worker, Natesh, introduces me to male and female sex workers who are soliciting for clients.

As we stand at one hotspot near a public park, chatting with some of the men and women, a client walks up to Natesh, and slaps him across the face, seizing his attention. After a bout of shouting, the other sex workers shoo the client away. Natesh appears unfazed by the incident: "he is very drunk... we try to avoid those types of clients because they are never wanting to wear condoms."

"And they take so long to go [ejaculate]," one of the other male sex workers chimes in.

"I am charging them extra if they take so long," another young guy says, grinning from ear to ear under his baseball cap.

"They can also be very violent to us, so we do not go with them," Natesh says, and with much conviction adds: "You see, we are more than just sex workers, we also have ideas for solving our own problems!" [Fieldnotes, March 2006]

These words, "...we also have ideas for solving our own problems!" was the moment that sparked a research collaboration with a community of male sex workers in Mysore, Karnataka. That same day Natesh also spoke candidly to me about his recent experiences with a quantitative study led by researchers based in Delhi. He said, "They asked me, 'What is your sexual identity? Do you practise sex work? Do you wear condoms? Are you HIV positive?' Then they took the information and we never heard back from them. I was left feeling very badly after this." I then asked Natesh and other community outreach workers whether they would be interested in leading a research process that would examine key issues that were of interest to them and generate information that they would own and could disseminate to other community members.

During an initial meeting that Natesh set up with community leaders to further discuss the potential for community research, some attendees hurled a few accusations at the Gates Foundation, one being that "Bill Gates is selling our blood." Research on idioms of blood stealing and selling cautions us against viewing such accusations either as mere misinterpretations, forms of resistance to post-colonial medical science, or as the wider consequences of global capitalism (Geissler 2005; Fairhead et al. 2006: 1111). But interestingly, community members did not denigrate the actual work of epidemiological surveillance practise. In fact, many expressed a desire to increase their participation in monitoring and evaluation processes. In particular, they wanted to be more actively involved in the integrated biological and behavioural assessment (IBBA), the findings of which were recognized as the most legitimate scientific evidence for assessing the progress of Avahan's interventions. External teams of biostatisticians located at the University of Manitoba, L'Université Laval, Imperial College London and the London School of Hygiene and Tropical Medicine, some of whom rarely stepped foot on Indian soil, took the lead in analyzing and interpreting the numerical data generated from the IBBA at a distance. The sex workers felt frustrated that their participation in the IBBA was limited to the identification of 'hotspots and to recruitment of fellow community members. One sex worker exclaimed during a local community meeting: "We want to explain what the numbers mean to our community!"

Indeed, sex workers felt strongly that they were left out of the process of interpreting the IBBA results. I came to understand the reiteration, "Bill Gates is selling our blood," as a local metaphor that spoke to their ambivalent and unequal positioning within Avahan's economy of evidence production, an economy that was also clearly reflected in the uneven disbursement of Avahan funds. Male sex workers privately commented to me on what they considered to be the extravagant living accommodations of some foreign academic beneficiaries of Gates Foundation grants in India and expressed criticism of the "international salaries" received by some Indian consultants closely tied to the foundation—monies which they felt would be better spent if they flowed through community-based organizations. Sex workers were acutely aware that an international enterprise had begun to flourish around the measurement of their bodies and behaviours, and also felt that monitoring and evaluation specialists maintained a monopoly over the interpretation of significant areas of their lives. Certainly sex workers were profoundly grateful to the Gates Foundation for the wealth of new specialized sexual health services available to their communities. However, they expressed that they wanted to increase their participation in evidence production activities, and in the following ways: by helping to re-word and re-order the IBBA survey questions, and by administering surveys to their community and interpreting what the numerical findings meant not only for HIV prevention but also financially, for the local sex work industry.

For these reasons, the sex work community expressed great enthusiasm with the idea of conducting a research project for and by their community. They claimed that it would be empowering to contribute directly to the information gathering process and the interpretation of findings. They decided that they wanted to focus the research study on identifying barriers to accessing health services for MSM due to high rates of HIV and STIs in this community and the low utilization of available health services (Reza-Paul et al. 2008). Furthermore, community leaders were clear that they wanted not only to generate information about why their community was reluctant to access health services; they also wanted to break down the barriers through community engagement in the research process itself. And so the participatory community research project began.

A training program was collaboratively developed that took into account the existing knowledge, skills, and experiences of the community leaders. Hired by the internationally renowned sex worker collective Ashodaya Samithi on a part-time basis, many of these leaders already possessed the skills to deliver safer sex information in "hard-to-reach locations"; and many had already participated in other kinds of research and knowledge creation activities in conjunction with Avahan's monitoring and evaluation activities.

The training project formally began in September 2006 with the formation of the community advisory committee comprising of MSM leaders from local community-based organizations serving MSM. The committee selected community researchers Community researchers to conduct the interviews: 10 who spoke and read Kannada, the local language; one individual who spoke Hindi; and three well-respected individuals who were selected to assist with the interview recruitment process. In an effort to access a diverse sample of participants, we chose interviewers who were connected to different social networks (according to age, cruising location frequented, and economic status).

On the first day of training, however, tension erupted between MSM leaders over their different organizational affiliations: some leaders were affiliated with organizations that were accused of ignoring the needs of male sex workers. Initially, two factions formed among the training participants and they were unwilling to sit at the same table. These political inflammations began to subside when an influential community leader implored everyone to consider the health needs of "the larger community," which included both men who have sex with men and male sex workers. The group decided that they needed a name to instil a sense of solidarity. "Adarsha" was chosen because of its positive meanings in the local language, Kannada: an icon, an idol, and a role model. Each time political tensions re-emerged, one of the team would announce "Adarsha!" to invoke group solidarity and defuse the tension.

The first day of training proceeded with an intensive session covering the cornerstone guidelines of ethical research: informed consent, coercion, confidentiality, and potential harm/benefits. On the second day, community researchers formulated recruitment procedures and were trained to approach members of their community using a recruitment script. It was stressed by Adarsha that the recruitment procedure must not disrupt sex work transactions or disturb clients and that research participants should be provided with a gift as a sign of appreciation for their time, as a sex worker who gives their time as an interview respondent may lose income. What intrigued me was how the workshop participants continually talked about how they could translate research ethical principles into the daily work they do. On one occasion, a participant indicated that the steps to research participant recruitment could double as an outreach recruitment strategy. Another participant claimed that he could utilize research recruitment procedures to pick up clients at cruising spots, a suggestion was that was met with much agreement and laughter by the rest of the workshop participants.

Prior to the training, two community leaders, with technical assistance from myself, formulated a tentative interview guide around the following key themes: stigma, sexual practise, harassment, health-seeking and protection behavior, and HIV knowledge. On the third day of training, Adarsha modified the question set by rewording questions that they felt would make their community feel uncomfortable. For instance, rather than asking about sex work directly, they advised that a more useful question would be to ask "have you ever given or received gifts in exchange for sex?" This became a crucial question for understanding the interactions between sex workers and their clients (Lorway et al. 2009). Adarsha also wanted the interviews to flow like a natural conversation so that the participants would feel comfortable talking about their experiences. To achieve this, Adarsha concluded that the question set must be worded in "kothi language" in order to break down the social distance maintained between "the researcher" and "the interviewee" during conventional research. The community researchers were trained on how to conduct a qualitative interview, which also served to pilot the interview guide. Pairs of community researchers practised the interviewing techniques they had learned. Then, each pair conducted mock interviews in front of the larger group, which provided constructive feedback.

The group described how they felt while being interviewed as a way to consider the ethical questions previously raised, resulting in further revisions to the interview guide. They discussed how probe techniques might relate to the ethical concern of coercion. In anticipation of a respondent becoming upset during an interview, probe questions would be limited or halted and information on free counselling resources available at Ashodaya would be provided. In line with the project goal of breaking down barriers to accessing health services through community engagement in the research process, the Adarsha team felt that it was important to correct any misinformation regarding HIV following an interview, at which time they would provide safer sex information pamphlets, condoms, and a description of Ashodaya health services.

For many of the male sex workers interviewed, this was the first time they had participated in qualitative research. Having previously participated in special bio-behavioural studies, however, some of the participants expressed to me that they were most pleased that they did not have to be pricked with a needle to withdraw blood for the qualitative study. One problem, however, did arise in the participatory project in relation to the sample size of the previous bio-behavioral surveillance studies. The community was accustomed to a much larger sample size, which meant that more people received the opportunity to participate in the study. Men who were not recruited into the qualitative study still showed up at the research site, insisting that they should be permitted to be interviewed. On a few occasions major shouting matches broke out between the participants who had not been selected for an interview and the community researchers who they recognized.

Although we tried to explain that qualitative studies only require a smaller number of research participants, their anger refused to subside. I asked the team if the problem related to the small gifts (like a tin lunch box worth a couple of US dollars) that we provided for other participants. The team insisted that the gift had less commercial value than the cost of the rickshaw that they took to the lodge. One community researcher said “the gift is too small anyway, and you can make much more from sex work in the time it takes to do an interview.” In talking to the annoyed individuals, I learned that being part of the research was a matter of honour, respect, and social inclusiveness—they had always been part of helping the community before through research, why were they excluded now? Thus community members regarded such large-scale evidence production as an important way that they exercised their political responsibilities and commitments to the community. In the end it was decided that in the name of maintaining relations of rapport with the community, the team would conduct the extra interviews.

Among the participants who agreed to be interviewed, their narrative included a commentary on how they felt about being interviewed by their peers, and the way that questions were worded by the community researchers.

> When I hear you speaking, I feel that you and I are the same. It is as though you have put a mirror to my own life.... You may be a person who has come to interview us for the project, but the way you are asking, with understanding of the hijras and with so much patience, it makes our heart lighter. I should thank you for that. [2o year old male sex worker]
>
> Now I'm revealing to you those facts that have been hidden deep inside my heart. Because you are also a male sex worker like me, that is why I like to tell.... [22 year old factory worker]

Once the interview concluded, many of the participants became quite emotional in expressing how the interview made them feel. Consistently, participants stated that a heavy weight had been lifted from them; most described the interview as providing a sense of relief from the burden of coping with stigma. This sentiment ran across the transcripts in statements such as "please ask me, I feel light hearted as I answer your questions." Indeed, most participants were pleased to answer questions.

Conversations generated during the interviews often continued into the "safe space," an adjoining room in the lodge where we stored our research materials, after the interview ended. There, sexual health information was exchanged and Ashodaya's services were outlined and promoted by the community researchers. On one occasion, an Adarsha member provided a personal account of how the clinic had helped clear up an infection in his genital region. On occasion I watched as the participants listened carefully to the community researchers and then requested to be taken to the clinic for a free health check-up.

This emotional response yielded an unexpected positive effect—a growing sense of social solidarity and relatedness. Following the interviewing and the public dissemination of the results back to the community, Adarsha established itself as an organization and its membership soon swelled to 400 members. Over time, the membership base continued to grow until it reached 2000 members. This emerging form of solidarity also became reflected in improved health-seeking behavior, almost immediately doubling the number of annual clinic attendees of men who have sex with men and hijras. As part of establishing Adarsha, the community researchers decided that they wanted to formally become a wing of Ashodaya Samithi, so that they could have access to Avahan-sponsored infrastructure to help support the achievement of their action plan. These goals included establishing specialized clinical services and drop-in centres for men who have sex with men and hijras in neighbouring *talukas* (sub-district units), which they did through Avahan's support.

Working closely alongside female sex worker allies, these goals were realized for both communities over the coming years (Argento et al. 2011; Dixon et al. 2012). They also stood prominently in public demonstrations, such as the June 2008 protest against the immoral trafficking prevention act (ITPA), and engaged with local and national news media.

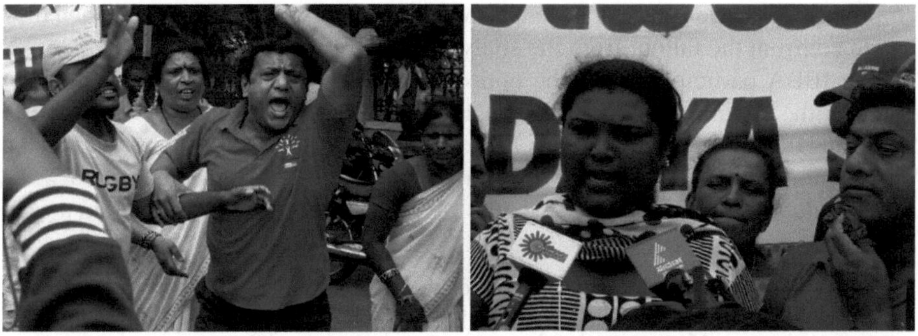

Over the coming years, members of Adarsha forcefully positioned their political interests in district- and state-level policy arenas, lobbying politicians to their cause. They even gained an audience with the Karnataka state Chief Minister and his ministerial council to address the social welfare and health concerns of hijras. Moreover, Adasha became an important player in the global alliance known as the Network of Sex Worker Projects and staged events to raise awareness of sex workers rights at international HIV conferences in the Asia Pacific region. Asserting their research training across local, state and international borders through numerous disseminations of their findings, Adasha increased their legitimacy within the Avahan programs. This was reflected in the opportunities that opened up for them to insert their input and participation within the Avahan's monitoring and evaluation procedures.

4.2 IBBA Fallout

The Integrated Biological and Behavioural Assessment (IBBA) is conducted only once every 2 or 3 years, but it is a major event in the life history of Avahan because of the scientific rigor it is assumed to embody. It is considered the golden standard of reliable monitoring and evaluation practises used to measure the major outcomes of Avahan's interventions. The findings from the IBBA are also prized because of the magnitude of the data set it has generated—56 assessments of high risk groups have been conducted in 29 districts across India's six high HIV prevalence states (ICMR and FHI 2011).

In 2007, the IBBA was conducted for the first time among men who have sex with men in five select districts of Karnataka. Because the Adarsha community research team had begun to prove their competency in conducting research, the monitoring and evaluation team—led by researchers from the l'Université Laval and the London School of Hygiene and Tropical Medicine—agreed to train the community researchers on how to administer the lengthy survey. The time location cluster sampling procedure also relied on their participation; for it requires the "random" identification of potential research participants from various hotspots. The Mysore team was excited by the new responsibilities they had acquired as co-producers of scientific evidence. However, their enthusiasm collapsed when they had to confront the fallout from the study results.

The IBBA participants had the option of receiving their HIV test results, and many of the community mobilizers decided to receive their diagnosis. The IBBA found an HIV prevalence of 23 % in Mysore city. Expressions of distress marked the faces of those who tested positive for HIV infection; their status confirmed when they eventually confided in me. One man who was planning to get married in a year, expressed his feelings of devastation:

> My family is not even knowing that I am doing sex work or that I am having sex with men … how can I tell them that I am a positive? Soon my parents are expecting me to be married, this year. My parents already want to start showing me different girls.

Some of these men, particularly those from agricultural communities surrounding the Mysore city proper, found themselves caught in a double bind. If they disclosed their status they feared that that they would not receive land owed to them as part of their family inheritance; they also believed they would be ostracized from their families for shaming them. On the other hand, if they did not disclose their status, they would be expected to get married to women and therefore risk infecting their partners, given the expectation of condomless sex in order to have children.

Over time, I watched as many of the HIV positive male sex workers ever more deeply invested their time and energy into their volunteer work at the CBO, and eventually they emerged as important leaders in the organization. Although the future support of their family was uncertain, the immediate social and economic ties they found at the CBO fostered a sense of obligation and service to the community.

As the years went by, male, female and transgender sex workers in Mysore channelled the energy surrounding the affective networks forming around HIV positive diagnoses following subsequent rounds of the IBBA. The CBO eventually set up a hospice for people who became sick with AIDS and established a wing in the parent sex worker organization for people living with HIV, known as Ashraya (Lazarus et al. 2012; Chevrier et al. 2015). As anthropologist Claudyne Chevrier and colleagues (2015) note, this new organization was well received by local people living with HIV. Even those who neither identified as a sex worker nor a sexual minority began to access the support and clinical services of this sex-worker run program because it was perceived, more generally, as providing non-discriminatory health services to people living with HIV (Chevrier et al. 2015). Importantly here, this HIV care and support program was neither initiated nor funded by Avahan. Thus, this example illustrates how the affective resonances and expanding networks of a community of people living with HIV could not be entirely contained by Avahan's program goals and success indicators. At the same time, this new project continued along the pathway set by Avahan, further prioritizing "health" as a means by which to frame the complex social struggles of this community.

4.3 The Tyranny of Community-Level Surveillance

Adarsha's parent organization, Ashodaya Samithi became a flagship program in India for two reasons, exemplifying "the success" claimed under Avahan. First, it represented an organization that was run by and for sex workers; and second, Ashodaya had shown some of the most dramatic reductions in curable STIs and HIV prevalence in India, which mathematical modellers tied to the community empowerment projects running there (Reza-Paul et al. 2008). Between 2010 and 2013, Avahan transitioned all of its community-centred intervention programs in India, like Ashodaya, to the public system, placing these interventions under the jurisdiction of the central government body, the National AIDS Control Organization (NACO), which flowed funds to the State AIDS Control Societies. Because of their recognized "results," NACO later funded Ashodaya to lead a total of ten district-level HIV interventions in the state of Karnataka.

During a visit with Ashodaya staff in October 2013, I was taken by Natesh to view a new HIV intervention that he was overseeing in Mandya, a district in South Karnataka known for its thriving sugarcane manufacturing industry. Natesh was proud of the new responsibility he had assumed in setting up and coordinating an HIV intervention. After arranging a vehicle to pick us up, Natesh instructed the driver to take us to a small taluka located just outside the Mandya city centre. Along the way Natesh informed me that a lot of men working at one of the sugar factories in this taluka had recently tested positive for HIV. During lunch breaks and after work, Natesh explained, some of the factory workers would congregate in the nearby bushes and have unprotected sex with local male sex workers. When we arrived at the taluka, a group of three community mobilizers were eagerly waiting to take us to the cruising area near the bushes to demonstrate how they had organized their intervention, and how they had strategically placed bags of condoms in trees and on some of the branches of the bushes. These outreach workers, who identified themselves to me as "MSWs" (male sex workers), explained how they worked through the social networks of their clients to "reach new MSM" on a daily basis, in order to register them into their programs. One community mobilizer said: "We are providing many different services to our clients; we are looking after their pleasure and their health." The small group began to laugh at the candid reference to sex work.

After my tour of this cruising spot, Natesh and the outreach workers escorted me into their community drop in centre in Mandya city. There, more than 20 community mobilizers were clustered together, sitting on the floor while trying to collate and consolidate all their tracking sheets, as it was the end of the month. Members of the group uttered their frustration around the new standardized tracking sheets that were imposed by NACO, which had now taken over the governance of HIV interventions in India from Avahan.

The complaints of the outreach workers ran along two directions: first they noted the difficulty of having to document highly sensitive information from new contacts on a daily basis (see Fig. 4.1); and second, they complained about the exorbitant

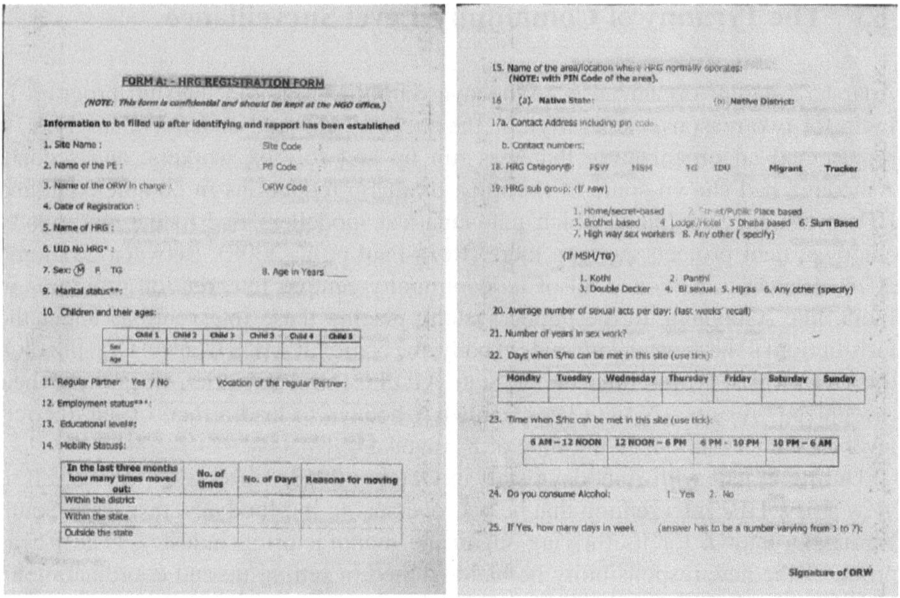

FORM A: - HRG REGISTRATION FORM

(NOTE: This form is confidential and should be kept at the NGO office.)

Information to be filled up after identifying and rapport has been established

1. Site Name : Site Code :
2. Name of the PE : PE Code :
3. Name of the ORW In charge : ORW Code :
4. Date of Registration :
5. Name of HRG :
6. UID No HRG* :
7. Sex: (M) F TG 8. Age in Years ____
9. Marital status**:
10. Children and their ages:

	Child 1	Child 2	Child 3	Child 3	Child 4	Child 5
Sex						
Age						

11. Regular Partner Yes / No Vocation of the regular Partner:
12. Employment status***:
13. Educational level#:
14. Mobility Status$:

In the last three months how many times moved out:	No. of times	No. of Days	Reasons for moving
Within the district			
Within the state			
Outside the state			

15. Name of the area/location where HRG normally operates:
(NOTE: with PIN Code of the area).

16 (a). Native State: (b) Native District:

17a. Contact Address including pin code

b. Contact numbers:

18. HRG Category®: FSW MSM TG IDU Migrant Trucker

19. HRG sub group: (If FSW)

1. Home/secret-based 2. Street/Public Place based
3. Brothel based 4 Lodge/Hotel 5 Dhaba based 6. Slum Based
7. High way sex workers 8. Any other (specify)

(If MSM/TG)

1. Kothi 2. Panthi
3. Double Decker 4. Bi sexual 5. Hijras 6. Any other (specify)

20. Average number of sexual acts per day: (last weeks' recall)
21. Number of years in sex work?
22. Days when S/he can be met in this site (use tick):

Monday	Tuesday	Wednesday	Thursday	Friday	Saturday	Sunday

23. Time when S/he can be met in this site (use tick):

6 AM – 12 NOON	12 NOON – 6 PM	6 PM - 10 PM	10 PM – 6 AM

24. Do you consume Alcohol: 1. Yes 2. No
25. If Yes, how many days in week (answer has to be a number varying from 1 to 7):

Signature of ORW

Fig. 4.1 Registration form filled out daily for new contacts

Section E Community Mobilisation			Oct-13	Nov-13	Dec-13	Jan-14	Feb-14	Mar-14		
e.1	# Meeting held at at Hotspot level	Report only the meetings held at site/Hotspot level								
e.2	# Community events held	Report only the Community event held in the month								
e.3	# cummulative SHG active	Report the cummunlative SHG so far								
e.3.1	#cummulative members in the SHG	Report the cummunlative members in the SHG so far								
e.4	# New SHG formed	Report only new SHG formed in the reporting month								
e.4.1	# Members in the SHG	Report only those members who are part of the new SHG								
e.5	Savings throug SHG	report total inidivual who so savings through the SHG								
e.6	No of Co-operative formed	if 2 or more Ti's together formed the co-operative head office Ti should report								
e.6.1	# Members in the Co-operative	Report how many membes get enrolled in Co-operative								
e.6.2	Monthly turn over of the co-operative	Report in Rupees the monthly turnover								
e.7	No of community members enrolled in CBO's(Cummulative)	Report how many membes are enrolled in CBO from the begining of CBO	Cummulative from (Till Sept-13)	Total Cummulative from Oct-13	Oct-13	Nov-13	Dec-13	Jan-14	Feb-14	Mar-14
			0	0						
e.7.1	No of community members enrolled in CBO's(New)	Report how many new membes are enrolled in CBO from the begining of CBO								
e.7.2	membership fee collected	Report in Rupees the monthly membership fees collected								
Section F Social Entitlement			Cummulative from (Till Sept-13)	Total Cummulative from Oct-13	Oct-13	Nov-13	Dec-13	Jan-14	Feb-14	Mar-14
f.1	No referred to Voter Identity Card(Cummulative)			0						
f.1.1	No received Voter Identity card(Cummulative)			0						
f.2	No referred to Ration Card (Cummulative)			0						
f.2.1	No received Ration card(Cummulative)			0						
f.3	No referred to Housing Schemes(Cummulative)			0						
f.3.1	No received Housing Schemes(Cummulative)			0						
f.4	No referred to Free Sites(Cummulative)			0						
f.4.1	No received Free Sites(Cummulative)			0						
f.5	No referred to Aadhar Card(Cummulative)			0						
f.5.1	No received Aadhar Card(Cummulative)			0						
f.6	No referred to Widow Pension(Cummulative)			0						
f.6.1	No received Widow Pension(Cummulative)			0						
Section G Trainings			Oct-13	Nov-13	Dec-13	Jan-14	Feb-14	Mar-14		
g.1	# Inhouse training conducted	In house training conducted to Peer educator,ORW in the reporting month								

Fig. 4.2 Monthly contact consolidation tracking sheet

time it took to actually compile the daily tracking sheets into the monthly forms (see Fig. 4.2). Natesh looked at me and said "it was not like this under Avahan. We were not required to fill out the community's personal information like this, and it is hard to get the number of contacts we need to show that we are doing good work when we have to ask for all this [personal] information." One of the community mobilizers interjected by saying "We are spending more time filling out forms now than actually spending time with our contacts in the field, giving them the condoms and information they need!" The murmur of complaints amidst the frenzied form filling continued, for hours.

How do we understand the embroilment of sex worker activists and health workers in these intensively bureaucratic activities? To what extent does the emphasis placed on "showing impact" through the production of quantitatively measurable evidence come to displace the interests of those participating in these interventions? The latter question echoes the concern of medical anthropologist Vincanne Adams (2013) in relation to the growing reliance in evidence-based global public health on statistical knowledge, which can "serve both a political function (in advocacy) and a depoliticizing function (by rendering social problems as 'objective facts')". To respond to the former question, I want to focus on two important moments in the life history of HIV interventions in India over the past decade: (1) The era of innovation, democratic participation, and the incitement to enumerate, and (2) The transition toward standardization, legibility, and centralized administration (2010–2013). I regard these two moments as important formative periods in the rise of a form of political domination that I refer to as the tyranny of community-level surveillance. In particular, I focus on the actual tracking sheets that outreach workers fill out – the types of documents that Annelise Riles (2006) has referred to as "artifacts of modern knowledge practises," and do so by paying particular attention to the aesthetics of the forms employed by outreach workers to meet the program targets of the reigning intervention regimes and the accountability requirements imposed by the government funder. As technologies of governance, I want to highlight the role that tracking sheets and other forms play in the re-inscription of particular modes of sovereignty, whereby tracking sheets serve as especially "dense transfer points" (Foucault) for the shifting power relations between sex workers, the nation state, and the transnationally-mediated advocacy networks.

4.4 The Era of Innovation, Democratic Participation, and the Incitement to Enumerate (2003–2010)

During this period, as mentioned in Chap. 3, Avahan funded and directly managed HIV interventions in six of India's high HIV prevalence states. Prior to Avahan, sexual minorities in India had encountered considerable exclusion from health and other social services (Cornish 2006). However, Avahan began to fund extensive specialized health services for sexual minorities in 2003, and promoted the

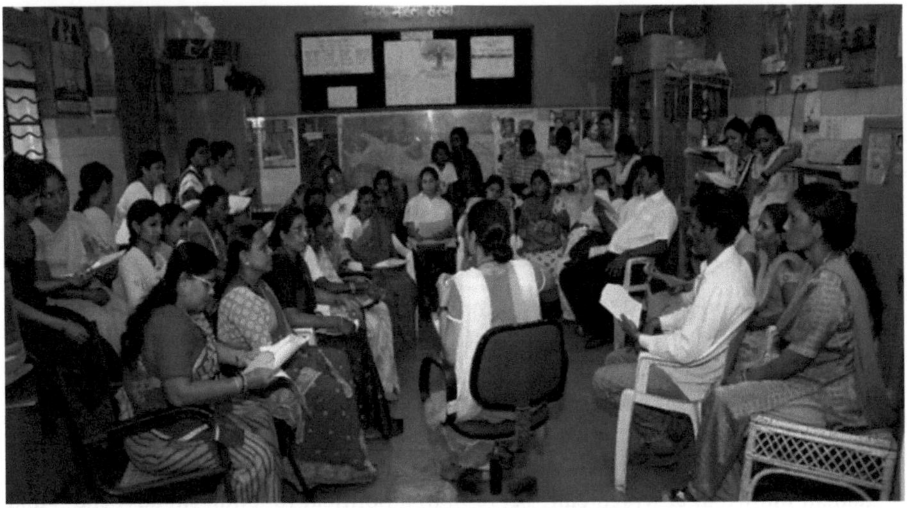

Fig. 4.3 Avahan promotional photo of sex workers and technical staff working together on a district level HIV intervention

destigmatization of sex workers (for example see "AIDS Sutra", Sen 2011) and people living with HIV/AIDS in India through the Hero's Project. Moreover, Avahan's community mobilization schemes helped to enhance the legitimacy of marginalized communities in the eyes of the Indian nation state, globally portraying Indian sex workers and sexual minorities in a positive light—performing activities for the greater good of society—as can be noted in the program promotional materials they published on their website (see Fig. 4.3).

One could argue that the resultant form of legitimacy is somewhat narrow in its confinement to HIV prevention, as it centred on the idea of an epidemic "concentrated" among male and female sex workers. Under the Avahan umbrella, diverse groups of sex workers and their transnational allies—including global rights activists, health promotion specialists, community workers, foreign academics, and local policy makers—mobilized around the idea of an epidemic "concentrated" among male and female sex workers to enhance the delivery of vital health resources to marginalized people. Nevertheless, despite the confinement to HIV-related health services, Avahan temporarily re-territorialized a sector of India's health system. By authorizing external experts to manage HIV prevention in six of India's states, access to specialized services for Indian citizens was, to some extent, governed at a supranational level.

As discussed in the last chapter, what is particularly striking about Avahan, was the explicit attempt to institute a business model to engage communities in HIV interventions:

> [Avahan] is primarily driven … by classic business principles: careful market segmentation (for instance, identifying and targeting the key groups involved in sex work), strategic alliances to achieve scale, and marketing, logistics, and distribution management....

> HIV control program implementation ... through the modus operandi of community mobilization ... requires a level of management focus that many programs to date have lacked. Providing a service to 20 people is one thing; reaching 200,000 requires management expertise.... Working at scale in this context implies both breadth and depth of intervention coverage, in other words, the saturation of the market with a quality product.
>
> Prevention services ... should be provided to all of the riskiest groups, geographically and typologically. This requires covering the locations where the epidemic is being fuelled and targeting all types of risk groups, including male and female sex workers, as well as intravenous drug users and their sexual partners. Depth means the provision of high-quality services through high-level technical input. This demands that intervention managers train local practitioners at the "grassroots" level, conduct site assessments, and engage in micro-level planning of daily outreach efforts to ensure high levels of rapport with the community. (Ramakrishnan and Alexander 2006)

Among the sex workers I collaborated with in Karnataka State, "community mobilization" appealed to them because of how this approach directly engaged them in evidence production. As outlined in the last chapter, based upon the mapping of "hotspots" and population-size estimates, public health practitioners set up networks of specialized clinics and drop-in centres near the hotspots where sex workers congregated for business, in order to attract them to the health services being offered. As part of the Avahan initiative, these "key populations" themselves were recruited to "mobilize" their peers, with the expectation that these marginalized people would become better connected to prevention and treatment services for HIV and sexually transmitted infections (STIs) (Verma et al. 2010). Explicitly abiding to a set of entrepreneurial logics, volunteer outreach workers were regarded as a "sales force" that would generate demand for clinical services in their community, thereby making the project sustainable (Ramakrishnan in Lorway 2013).

My ethnographic work revealed how these outreach workers spent considerable time trying to reach their daily contact targets, filling out spread sheets with the support of program staff. At weekly "community guide meetings" I witnessed how tracking forms served as heuristic devices that allowed sex workers to characterize what was happening in the field. Comparing and pooling tracking information between themselves enabled them to quickly pinpoint a part of the city where police violence impeded their health service delivery, or where a gang of goondas [violent gangs of men] were disrupting outreach work. So indeed these tracking forms served as technologies that quickly sparked politicizations around health services utilization problems, enabling sex workers to strategize and re-focus their energies when it came to outreach work in the field.

What was also intriguing during this period was how there was a proliferation of various versions of tracking sheets throughout India, across the "high prevalence states" in which Avahan worked. In Fig. 4.4 you will notice a very small sample of the multitude of differently designed forms used to keep track of contacts and other outreach activities in the States of Andhra Pradesh, Maharashtra, Karnataka, and Tamil Naidu. The latitude to develop these somewhat unique tracking forms was conditioned by the reigning Avahan business model advanced by Ashok Alexander and AparjitaRamakrisnan, particularly the component of "flexibility," which permits and even encourages interveners to take some "reasonable risks" to address

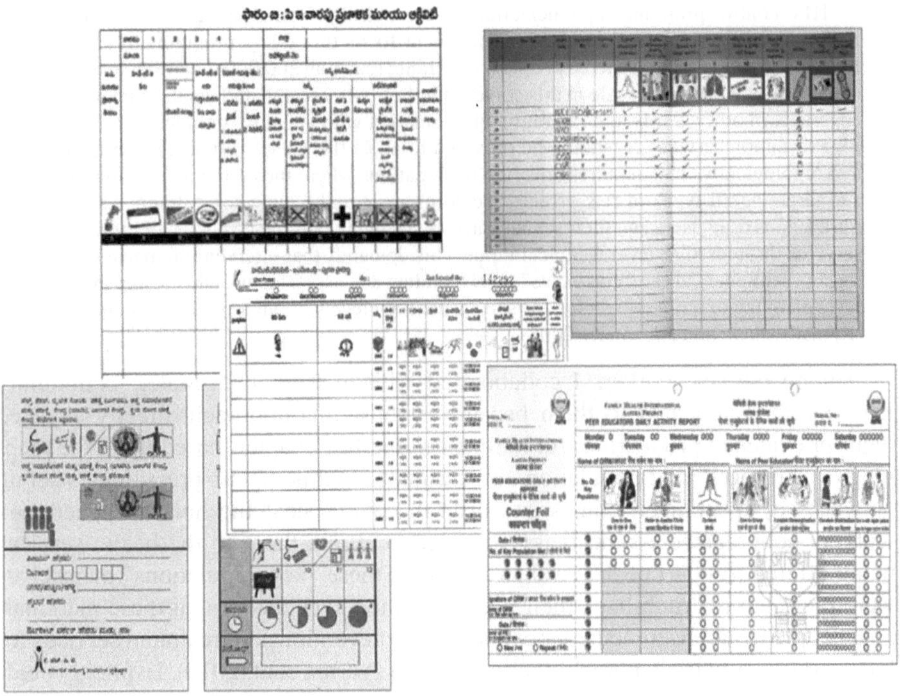

Fig. 4.4 Regional variations in outreach tracking forms (designed to be user friendly for sex workers) in Andhra Pradesh, Maharashtra, Karnataka, and Tamil Naidu

on-the-ground challenges, so long as the effects are carefully measured in relation to outcomes.

> Flexibility: Market solutions are constantly evolving and lasting business adapt with them. Avahan is trying things for the first time, placing large and small bets. Avahan trusts its own judgment, take reasonable risks, check results, and make technically appropriate changes as the realities on the ground demand. (Alexander and Ramakrishana 2006)

Indeed the entrepreneurial ethic of innovation was a key driving force in the production of these different types of forms in this era. Seeing themselves as being in competition with each other, district-level interventions creatively designed their own tracking sheets to best capture data around Avahan's prefixed indicators of success. In fact, many of the sex workers I worked with spoke of this "healthy competition" as being good for HIV prevention, for it encouraged districts to even exceed their "population coverage targets."

Some of these tracking sheets contain visual images, so that even illiterate outreach workers can record quantitative information. Moreover it should be noted that the design of tracking forms in this era was developed in close consultation with leaders from the sex work community. Although these forms ultimately gathered information around a common set of prefixed quantitative indicators, the actual design and form of these tracking sheets often developed through a democratic consultative process involving local health promotion staff, academic researchers, and sex workers. Many of the sex workers I worked with expressed great pride in the unique strategies their teams had employed to enumerate their outreach activities, sometimes using smaller notepads to discreetly capture information before it was later transferred to the forms.

The fostering of creativity around the design and deployment of tracking forms in this era exemplifies what Ari Samsky (2012) terms as "scientific sovereignty"; for the proliferation of innovative tracking sheets ultimately flows from the mix of epidemiological and entrepreneurial discourses deployed by Avahan's transnational consortium of health scientists, business managers, and local program directors (Lorway and Khan 2014). Although NACO, as the central government HIV policy body certainly wielded ultimate authority over scientists and program mangers working on Avahan sites, NACO directly answered to the national health minister at the time, closely consulted with Avahan officials and, as such, avoided the tangled bureaucratic web of Ministry of Health and Family Welfare. Therefore, Avahan's program implementation was granted considerable leeway to organize and channel resources for specialized services at the grassroots level with seemingly minimal bureaucratic interference or regulation from state- or district-level Indian government officials (Samsky 2012:317).

While this period of "incitement to enumerate" can be associated with the positive health outcomes yielded under Avahan, the central edict of gathering evidence that could eventually be mathematically modelled to show intervention progress created contradictions in terms of reaching some segments of populations of men who have sex with men and leaving out others. As we saw in the last chapter, in the three urban sites where I worked, certain cruising spots frequented by transgender devotees to the goddess Yellamma, masculine-acting men who did not assume a same sex sexual identity, and drug using male sex workers were avoided as these groups were viewed as being "un-mobilizable." Tracking sheets could not be readily filled out for these groups, for many of them had neither fixed addresses, nor were they willing to provide cell phone numbers. As a result, not only were important opportunities for epidemic prevention overlooked but these zones of exclusion were rendered invisible beneath the larger picture of success painted by Avahan's monitoring and evaluation specialists and based on the selective form filling practises of community mobilizers.

4.5 The Transition Toward Standardization, Legibility, and Centralized Administration (2010–2013)

Between 2010 and 2013, Avahan transitioned all of its community-centred intervention programs in India to the public system, placing these interventions under the jurisdiction of the State AIDS Control societies (Rao 2010; Sgaier et al. 2013). As Avahan's managerial infrastructure transitioned, criticism of the program as a lavishly over-funded intervention came to a head. Controversies erupted over how the public system could sustain the successes demonstrated by the Avahan-supported infrastructure of specialized clinical services and community mobilization activities. Because district and state–level health system officials had hitherto been largely shut out of Avahan's operation, heated questions unfurled around the capacity of the public system to take over the HIV initiative.

In 2003, the target set for community mobilization by Avahan had been that 50 % of CBOs run by sex workers would take over targeted interventions in India. However, only a much smaller fraction of CBOs were regarded by the state as being prepared to assume leadership in 2010, as Avahan's "success" was not evenly distributed across India. During the transition period, consultants working for the National AIDS Control Organization assessed a number of local NGOs and community-based organizations as being unfit to assume leadership over targeted interventions in their district, and they had their funding pulled.

The downgrading of many frontline organizations throughout India came in tandem with NACO's execution of increasingly intrusive and coercive modes of surveillance. New tracking sheets were introduced which were more standardized, being designed to gather more personal information, and taking considerably more time to complete. Gone were the opportunities for the creation of diverse tracking sheets that were tailored to speak to the specificity of local communities and the uneven literacy levels among individuals. Eclipsing Avahan's previously reigning discourse of innovation, entrepreneurialism and democratic participation, this shift on the part of the Indian State pointed to the thin and temporary nature of the modes of scientific sovereignty enacted under Avahan.

The various transnational-mediated collectives that assembled under the Avahan banner rose to challenge the increasingly draconian policies of NACO. The following excerpt from a publically released draft letter, composed by the National Network of Sex Workers, the Indian Harm Reduction Network, the Lawyers Collective HIV/AIDS Unit, and the Integrated Network for Sexual Minorities, illustrate something of the turbulence that swirled around the state's deployment of intrusive monitoring and evaluation techniques, which accompanied coercive HIV testing, to govern India's "most-at-risk populations":

> The inability to meet testing targets leads to a negative evaluation by the Technical Surveillance Unit (TSU) and/or State AIDS Control Society (SACS), triggering a series of adverse consequences….
>
> Some targeted interventions (TIs) are reportedly organising 'health camps' to test persons with no reported high risk behavior in order to fill in numbers of people tested for HIV.

The letter continues by criticizing NACO's implementation of mandatory standardized "line-listing" forms:

> Project staff in TIs are mandated to record the name, address and other contact information of MARPs and share this data with TSU/SACS…. We would like to reiterate that respecting client confidentiality is not only a legal requirement but also a good public health strategy, as it improves attendance at clinics, enables clients' to reveal medical or related risks and facilitates correct diagnosis and treatment.

Despite the objections raised by civil society networks, NACO's standardized line-listing forms came to rule India's geography of HIV intervention. However, the highly coordinated effort to produce "sound" measurable evidence on the art of the Indian government, actually dismisses any recognition of how local attempts to subvert this coercive mode of sovereignty may actually undermine HIV prevention, testing and treatment efforts, as the fake testing camps demonstrate.

More recently, in March 2015, I conducted a focus group with community leaders in Mysore; one male sex worker remarked:

> During Avahan, the whole canvass was ours for developing programs. It was created with a social cause, serving for the community. Now it is like company work. The government program is thinking like a TI [targeted intervention], like a science; but we are thinking like a group. Even I have started thinking like a project person ... how can I stick to this job. *Now* the focus is on form filling, not what is happening in the field. How perfect can I do the document? If the paper is ok that is enough. Because when the government [officials from the State AIDS Control society] comes to evaluate us, they only want to see the documents, they don't do follow-up with the community in the field like they did in Avahan. This is why so many organizations are just filling up the forms, *to fill them up*—just so they can keep their funding ... which is understandable. But this is not good.

This quotation points to the role the aesthetics of tracking forms play in the art of governing sex workers for HIV prevention. The creativity and innovation of "community friendly" tracking forms inspired during the Avahan era eventually gave way to a more rigid and time consuming reporting process, one which resembles the slower reporting systems in other Indian government-sponsored health programs. In August 2014, the National AIDS Control Organization (NACO), which once had considerable autonomy to consult with Avahan's consortia of international experts and enact swift policy changes, was merged with the Ministry of Health and Family Welfare—a move that was met with condemnation by sexual rights activists across India who fear a return to the highly stigmatizing conditions surrounding health services provision that existed prior to the Avahan initiative.

Although I have tried to show some of the transformations around the governance of HIV prevention in India by dividing important moments into two epochs, these transformations should not be conceptualized merely as a shift between two different or separate systems of governance—from an "innovative and democratic" one to a system that is "older," plodding, and entangled in bureaucratic "red tape" (Gupta 2012). Rather, I would argue that these two reporting systems articulate intimately with each other. The period of "incitement" supported by Avahan—a program that was authorized and regulated by NACO through various direct and indirect modes of rule—was crucial for how the modern post-colonial Indian State apparatus operated to enlarge its bureaucratic territory to engulf dissenting social movements: first by effectively "outsourcing" a large sector of the health system to a transnational consortia of experts; and second, by reining in and harnessing the (sometimes unruly) "creative" community engagements and affective investments that this outsourcing later generated.

References

Adams, V. (2013). Evidence-based global public health. In J. Biehl & A. Petryna (Eds.), *When people come first* (pp. 54–90). Princeton: Princeton University Press.

Argento, E., Reza-Paul, S., Lorway, R., Jain, J., Bhagya, M., Fathima, M., Sreeram, S. V., Hafeezur, R. S., & O'Neil, J. (2011). Confronting structural violence in sex work: Lessons from a community-led HIV prevention project in Mysore, India. *AIDS Care, 23*(1), 69–74.

Chevrier, C., Khan, S., Reza-Paul, S., & Lorway, R. (2015). 'No one was there to care for us': Ashodaya Samithi's community-led care and support for people living with HIV in Mysore, India. *Global Public Health, 11*(4), 1–14.

Cornish, F. (2006). Challenging the stigma of sex work in India: Material context and symbolic change. *Journal of Community & Applied Social Psychology, 16*(6), 462–471.

Cornwall, A., & Jewkes, R. (1995). What is participatory research? *Social Science & Medicine, 41*(12), 1667–1676.

Dixon, V., Reza-Paul, S., D'Souza, F. M., O'Neil, J., O'Brien, N., & Lorway, R. (2012). Increasing access and ownership of clinical services at an HIV prevention project for sex workers in Mysore, India. *Global Public Health, 7*(7), 779–791.

Fairhead, J., Leach, M., & Small, M. (2006). Where techno-science meets poverty: Medical research and the economy of blood in The Gambia, West Africa. *Social Science & Medicine, 63*(4), 1109–1120.

Geissler, P. W. (2005). 'Kachinja are coming!': Encounters around medical research work in a Kenyan village. *Africa, 75*(02), 173–202.

Gupta, A. (2012). *Red tape: Bureaucracy, structural violence, and poverty in India.* Durham: Duke University Press.

Indian Council of Medical Research and FHI. (2011). *Integrated Behavioral and Biological Assessment (IBBA): Guidelines for surveys of populations at risk of HIV infection.* New Delhi: Indian Council of Medical Research and FHI. http://www.fhi360.org/sites/default/files/media/documents/Integrated%20Behavioral%20and%20Biological%20Assessment%20Guidelines%20for%20Surveys%20of%20Populations%20at%20Risk%20of%20HIV%20Infection.pdf.

Israel, B., Eng, E., Schulz, A., & Parker, E. (2005). Introduction to methods in CBPR for health. In *Methods in community-based participatory research for health* (pp. 3–26). San Francisco: Jossey-Bass.

Lazarus, L., Reza-Paul, S., Pasha, A., Jairam, S., Hafeez Ur Rahman, S., O'Neil, J., & Lorway, R. (2012). Exploring the role of community-based peer support in improving access to care and antiretroviral treatment for sex workers in Mysore, India. *Journal of HIV/AIDS & Social Services, 11*(2), 152–168.

Lorway, R. (2013). How to exit an epidemic: Philanthrocapitalism, community mobilization, and the domestication of Sexual Dissidence in South India. In R. A. Smith (Ed.), *Global HIV/AIDS politics, policy, and activism, persistent challenges and emerging issues (Volume 3: Activism and community mobilization)* (Vol. 3, p. 203e222). New York: Praeger Press.

Lorway, R., & Khan, S. (2014). Reassembling epidemiology: Mapping, monitoring and making-up people in the context of HIV prevention in India. *Social Science & Medicine, 112*, 51–62.

Lorway, R., Reza-Paul, S., & Pasha, A. (2009). On becoming a male sex worker in Mysore: Sexual subjectivity,"empowerment", and community-based HIV prevention research. *Medical Anthropology Quarterly*, *23*(2), 142–160.

Lorway, R., Thompson, L. H., Lazarus, L., du Plessis, E., Pasha, A., Fathima Mary, P., Khan, S., & Reza-Paul, S. (2014). Going beyond the clinic: Confronting stigma and discrimination among men who have sex with men in Mysore through community-based participatory research. *Critical Public Health, 24*(1), 73–87.

Lupton, D. (1995). *The imperative of health: Public health and the regulated body* (Vol. 90). London: Sage Publications.

Ramakrishnan, A., & Alexander, A. (2006). Practicing theory: Management in HIV intervention. *Harvard International Review, 28*(2), 58.

Rao, P. J. (2010). Avahan: The transition to a publicly funded programme as a next stage. *Sexually Transmitted Infections, 86*(Suppl 1), i7–i8.

Reza-Paul, S., Beattie, T., Syed, H. U., Venukumar, K. T., Venugopal, M. S., Fathima, M. P., Raghavendra, H. R., et al. (2008). Declines in risk behaviour and sexually Transmitted infection prevalence following a community-led HIV preventive intervention among female sex workers in Mysore, India. *AIDS, 22*(Suppl 5), S91–S100.

Riles, A. (2006). *Documents: Artifacts of modern knowledge*. Ann Arbor: University of Michigan Press.

Samsky, A. (2012). Scientific sovereignty: How international drug donation programs reshape health, disease, and the state. *Cultural Anthropology, 27*(2), 310–332.

Sen, A. (2011). *AIDS Sutra: Untold stories from India*. New York: Anchor.

Sgaier, S. K., Ramakrishnan, A., Dhingra, N., Wadhwani, A., Alexander, A., Bennett, S., Bhalla, A., Kumta, S., Jayaram, M., Gupta, P., & Piot, P. K. (2013). How the Avahan HIV prevention program transitioned from the Gates Foundation to the government of India. *Health Affairs, 32*(7), 1265–1273.

Verma, R., Shekhar, A., Khobragade, S., Adhikary, R., George, B., Ramesh, B. M., Ranebennur, V., Mondal, S., Patra, R. K., Srinivasan, S., & Vijayaraman, A. (2010). Scale-up and coverage of Avahan: A large-scale HIV-prevention programme among female sex workers and men who have sex with men in four Indian states. *Sexually Transmitted Infections, 86*(Suppl 1), i76–i82.

Part III
Kenya: Bioexperimentalization

Chapter 5
A South-to-South Collaboration

Abstract As Avahan began to transition to the public system in 2010, the Gates Foundation began a concerted effort to "transfer the lessons learned" from HIV interventions in India to Kenya, through what was referred to as a "South-to-South collaboration." This project translated into the bi-directional travel, between Bangalore and Nairobi, of Indian, Kenyan, and Canadian health scientists, along with allied program managers, government health officials, and leaders from the communities most highly affected by the HIV epidemic. In this chapter, some of the tensions that emerged within the context of this instance of south-to-south collaboration are examined, first by looking at what happened when the people—groups of scientist, program managers, health officials and community leaders—travelled between India and Kenya. Then it is discussed how the enumerative techniques that migrated from India articulated with a longer history of biomedical research in Kenya, merging administrative, business and epidemiology, with bio-experimental logics in the management of routine sexual health service delivery to sex workers.

Keywords HIV prevention • Kenya • Biomedical research • Men who have sex with men • Male sex workers

As Avahan began to transition to the public system in 2010, the Gates Foundation began a concerted effort to "transfer the lessons learned" from Avahan to Kenya, through what was referred to as a "South-to-South collaboration." This project translated into the bi-directional travel, between Bangalore and Nairobi, of Indian, Kenyan, and Canadian health scientists, along with allied program managers, government health officials, and leaders from the communities most highly affected by the HIV epidemic.

A constellation of enumerative technologies—designed to make "sexual risk" visible, knowable and measureable, in standardized terms—also moved across these national boundaries, primarily in the direction from India to Kenya. These included (1) the typological approaches used to identify "the most at risk populations"; (2) the geographic mapping techniques that calculate the number, time, and location of "hotspots" to determine where and when sex workers and sexual minorities congregate to find sexual partners; (3) the community mobilization schemes, which utilize the mapping data to form a blueprint for outreach activities; and (4) the daily tracking forms, which serve as a community-level program monitoring system.

R. Lorway, *AIDS Activism, Science and Community Across Three Continents*,
Social Aspects of HIV 1, DOI 10.1007/978-3-319-42199-5_5

Paralleling India's geography of intervention, the emergent enumerative regime in Nairobi, which instituted new standards for counting people and places in need of service delivery, significantly contributed to the "making up" of identities, communities, and localities as the intervention terminologies and concomitant logics began to proliferate and become socially embedded (Sangaramoorthy and Benton 2012). Shortly following my first visit to Nairobi in 2010, Indian, Kenyan and Canadian health scientists initiated a large multi-province mapping of most "at risk populations" (female and male sex workers and MSM) throughout Kenya. Sex workers who participated in the mapping as field team enumerators or key informants soon began uttering the lexicon of the mapping project, referring to their fellow members as "MARPS." Within a year, however, health scientists and program planners began to replace the term "MARPS" with "key populations" based on the critical feedback of leaders from the affected communities who refused the term on the grounds that it was re-stigmatizing.

During a discussion of research participant sampling in the context of a qualitative research training session I coordinated with a group of female and male sex workers, those who had been exposed to the mapping training readily recited the new typological scheme for sex work, a scheme constructed during the course of the geographic mapping study and based on notions of place (e.g., street-based, sex den-based, bar-based, home-based, internet-based, and so on). However, the arrival of these new technical standards for delivering health services was not always well received by those utilizing the resources. Sex workers and sexual minorities alike often resisted, subverted, and "re-assembled" them in ways that were not always expected by the scientists who invented the standards.[1]

In this chapter, I examine some of the tensions that emerged within the context of this instance of south-to-south collaboration, first by looking at what happened when the people—groups of scientist, program managers, health officials and community leaders—travelled between India and Kenya. Then I discuss how the enumerative techniques that migrated from India articulated with a longer history of biomedical research in Kenya, merging administrative, business and epidemiology, with bio-experimental logics in the management of routine sexual health service delivery to sex workers. This background is necessary for understanding how HIV surveillance procedures in Nairobi began to transform the very ground on which local sex workers realized AIDS activism and other social justice projects, a point that will be examined in the final chapter.

5.1 Postcolonial Tensions

Beginning in 2010, groups of Kenyan scientists (mostly medical microbiologists), mid-level health officials, program managers, and members from sex worker CBOs travelled to Bangalore and Mysore to view the workings of HIV programs there. Presenting "community mobilization" as the cornerstone of Avahan programs, the

[1] Lampland and Star (2009) make a similar point in their essay *Beyond the Human Standard?*.

local Indian team took the visiting Kenyan groups for various "field visits" to the cruising spots where sex workers and sexual minorities congregated to meet their sexual partners, so that the Kenyans could inspect how the enthusiastic outreach workers were greeting contacts, filling out their tracking forms, and eventually collating their data with program managers.

Viewing these programs elicited different responses among the visitors, which I learned about through my informal conversations on their return to Kenya. Kenyan scientists and clinicians were particularly struck by the meagre STI testing resources available in India. Unlike CDC/PEPFAR-funded sex worker clinics in Kenya, which supported laboratory testing for syphilis, Chlamydia, and gonorrhoea as well as HIV, sex worker clinics in India only provided presumptive therapy and syndromic management without regular STI lab confirmation (except for the IBBA).[2] The Kenyan scientists were, however, deeply impressed by how "community mobilization" had created loyal and regular health service users. Kenyan government health officials and program managers seemed to find most remarkable the wide "coverage" of the sex worker populations and the way that outreach activities effectively connected sex workers to health services, even reaching the most "hidden" and "hard-to-reach" locations. Sex workers from two community-based organizations in Nairobi were also profoundly impressed by the way Indian sex workers appeared to be "taking the lead in India."

During the same time period, similar groupings of Indian and Canadian scientists (mostly epidemiologists and demographers), health officials, program managers and community members involved in the Avahan program began visiting Kenya. Those I spoke with formulated a number of critical observations of their programs. Although greatly impressed by the STI clinical resources available to the Kenya clinicians—which included a level 3 containment laboratory at Kenyatta Hospital—the Indian and Canadian scientists strongly disapproved of the sex worker interventions, as one Indian scientist told me: "The Kenya programs are just too biomedical—more needs to be done to create enabling environments for sex workers. This needs to happen outside the clinic!" Indian and Canadian scientists together generally agreed with the criticism of the Kenyan interventions as being "too biomedical," given how the programs were indeed centred around meeting the demands of clinical indicators—that is, delivering biological targets to CDC/PEPFAR through sex worker cohorts studies (a form of longitudinal research that has been important for establishing and maintaining the long and distinguished careers of the Kenya and Canadian medical microbiologists). "Unlike ours in India," one Indian program manager said, "the Kenyans don't really have the same community drop-in centres at most of these clinics… where sex workers can share their common experiences." One of the Indian sex workers similarly expressed their disproval by adding "Even the clinic receptionist is 'non-community!'" A more senior program director from India further explained the contrast to me "[The sex worker clinics in

[2]Presumptive STI therapy involves providing group of people assumed to be at high risk with medications (antibiotics) without lab testing and regardless of whether they present symptoms such as lesions, sores or discharge. Syndromic management involves treating "high risk groups" only when they present with STI symptoms (based on visual diagnosis or narrative of painful urination, etc., but is practiced without laboratory testing).

Nairobi] do have community mobilizers like us but theirs are only accountable to the clinic and not to the community. They don't understand how community mobilization is really supposed to be run."

To understand the contrasting approaches to delivering health services to sex workers in India versus Kenya, it is helpful to look to the specific local histories of collaboration and the human resources mobilized for their respective interventions. For program implementation, which was explicitly framed according to business logics, Avahan primarily drew its human resources from the social services and economic development sector in India, when it began work in 2003. Kenya's longer history of sex worker programs and HIV control, since the early 1980s, relied upon the academic collaborations between Canadian, Kenyan, and US medical microbiologists. A number of the Kenyan scientists, I should add, received their advanced training in microbiology at the Universities of Manitoba and Washington (Krotz 2012; Geissler 2011; Booth 2004). If the health service delivery model for Avahan was best portrayed in the figure of "the community outreach worker" who serves as the "the sales force" that creates and sustains community demand for health services, then the Kenyan model of health service delivery was exemplified by "the cohort study" and "the clinical trial." Reinforcing this biomedical orientation, a crowded landscape of HIV funders (such as the International AIDS Vaccine Initiative (IAVI), the US Centers for Disease Control (CDC), both with offices based in Nairobi, along with the Kenyan Medical Research Institute (KEMRI) and the Kenyan AIDS Vaccine Initiative (KAVI)) financed the network of North American and Kenya scientists conducting ongoing clinical research.

Heated disagreement broke out as a flurry of comparisons was drawn between Indian and Kenya HIV interventions. The Gates Foundation, taking the advice of the Canadian scientists, eventually decided that key program managers from India should be stationed in Nairobi to form a technical support unit, which would advise the government on how to create standardized monitoring systems to measure program coverage. This objective of the technical support unit also included the programs under the jurisdiction of the Kenyan scientists. In 2010, representatives from the Gates Foundation Headquarters in Seattle made their way to Nairobi to begin negotiations with Kenyan government health officials while the Indian program managers, soon hired into positions on the technical support unit, began to hold meetings with government officials to plan how they could collaborate in the South-to-South project. Kenyan Health officials welcomed the resources that the technical support unit had to offer, and these officials soon became co-investigators on grants with investigators from the University of Manitoba, eventually sharing co-authorship on publications, and receiving sitting fees and honoraria for attending meetings that took place outside their governmental offices. However, for many of the clinical scientists who previously had free reign over their clinical research with sex workers, the arrival of Indian program managers who took up residence on Kenyan soil was met with some hostility. One Kenyan health scientist exclaimed in front of his colleagues one day "We are not taking orders from these Indians. We have already dealt with this problem [during] colonialism." These postcolonial stirrings spoke rather explicitly to the history that Sana Aiyar (2015) details with respect to how

Indians came to form "the administrative and economic middle classes" in Kenya under British colonial rule. Important to note here, is how the role of "the West" more generally is omitted in both parts of the colonial-postcolonial continuity evoked by the Kenyan scientist.

The interactions between sex workers in India and Kenya were marked by much less tension. Indian female and male sex worker leaders from the Ashodaya Samithi collective, who were officially listed as co-investigators (as "knowledge users") on the CIHR-funded HIV vaccine acceptability research program I was leading, made contact with local sex work leaders in Nairobi through the recently mobilized activist network known as the Kenyan Sex Worker's Alliance. The encounter between the two groups of male and female sex workers was so positive that Ashodaya extended an invitation for them to visit Mysore, to view their programs.

During the boycott of the international AIDS Conference in Washington DC in 2012, a parallel session organized by transnational networks such as the global Network of Sex Work Projects (NSWP) was held in Kolkata.[3] There, John Mathenge, the director of HOYMAS (Health Options for Young Men on HIV/AIDS/STI), a male sex worker collective based in a working class neighborhood in Nairobi, connected with Ashodaya Samithi and, following the boycott demonstration, travelled to Mysore to view their programs. In speaking with the director he expressed how amazed he was to see the community "running the programs." Mathenge was particularly impressed by the influence Ashodaya exerted over clinical services. Through a clinic management committee they had formed, Ashodaya advised the clinicians on the respectful treatment of sex workers (also see Dixon et al. 2012). He was also taken with the community research projects we had conducted over the years in Mysore. After his return to Kenya, John approached me with the idea of doing a similar life history project, in collaboration with Ashodaya, so that the questions, data collection, interpretations and recommendations would be driven by the experiences, interests and insights of the male sex worker community in Nairobi. I agreed.

At the same time, a Kenya scientist who was running a male sex worker cohort study operating at one of the sex worker's clinics in Nairobi approached me to discuss the profound health problems facing the participants enrolled in his study. As the medical microbiologist explained, between 2009 and 2010, the 510 STI clinic

[3] Sex workers and people who use drugs along with their allies held two side meetings to protest the choice to have the 2012 International AIDS conference in Washington, D.C, USA because of non-immigrant visa prohibitions imposed for these two groups. Visa applicants were expected to respond to the following questions: (1) Are you or have you ever been a drug abuser or drug addict? (2) Are you coming to the United States to engage in prostitution or unlawful commercialized vice or have you been engaged in prostitution or procuring prostitutes within the past 10 years? An affirmative response would render the applicant ineligible. Although the US law render people living with HIV ineligible for a visa was repealed under the Obama administration, sex workers and people using drugs, who comprise two groups who are highly susceptible to HIV infection, remained ineligible for a US entry visa or visa waiver. In July 2012, the global sex work activist community held a side meeting in Kolkata while a group of protesters championing the rights of communities of people using drugs assembled in Kiev. Both events received funding support from the international AIDS society.

attendees showed a baseline HIV prevalence of 40 % and an annual HIV incidence among those uninfected of 12 %. He was understandably exasperated as he told me how they had provided condoms and lubricants, counselling, and HIV prevention education—yet the sero-conversion rate was still so high. He reached out to me with the expectation that I could somehow help them to explore what they were missing, something "social" or "structural" that was happening "outside the clinic."[4] I approached Mathenge with the idea of combining both projects, and he enthusiastically endorsed this collaboration. Both Mathenge and the microbiologist became co-investigators on the eventual research project, funded by the Canadian Institutes of Health Research, while I was listed as the principal investigator. In short, we made the agreement that the quantitative behavioural survey would build on the knowledge generated by the life histories produced by a team of community researchers. What resulted from this research collaboration brought together sex workers from Kenya and India with local health scientists and program planners from the technical support unit in a "south-to south" study (the S2S study), a project operating under the assumption that there were also important "community lessons" and wisdom that could be shared between India and Kenya.

5.2 "What's Your Denominator?"

Our community researcher training sessions took place in the same space occupied by the technical support unit, in the Geomaps office building located in Upperhill, Nairobi. Because the funding for the technical support unit and the S2S study flowed from the same location in Canada (the University of Manitoba, that is), the training venue was convenient for paying participants their daily travel per diems, as a financial officer was stationed there. This office space, where the technical support unit was located, was also home to a new NGO that the University of Manitoba set up to provide on-the-ground administrative support to research projects and to be eligible to receive foreign funding for projects that required a "local" partner organization. This practise has become fairly common among Western academic health research units. Donors, however, are certainly aware of this practise and usually build in budget requirements that restrict how much funds can be paid out to western institutions to ensure that the bulk of funds are spent "in country."[5]

---

[4] Although the group of medical micro biologists under the lead of Frank Plummer were planning to put in a grant to CIHR, they asked if I would put in a separate grant that would explore the social and structural dimensions of the HIV vulnerability of male sex workers. They realized that the "problem of rapid sero-conversaion" went well beyond the clinic.

[5] This became clear to me during my grant review work for the research granting organization known as Evidence for HIV prevention in Southern Africa (EHPSA), which is an initiative funded by UKAID and SIDA. Donors reviewing the grant applications with those of us representing different forms of scientific expertise queried how "local" some NGOs were. Proposal budget that showed the majority of funds trickling back to foreign universities were requested to revise their budget to show more funds staying in country.

One day, following a training session, a member of the technical support unit raised the issue of "denominators," as he approached me with a concerned look. He began to show me a landscape view of a graph on his laptop that presented a series of bar diagrams, ranking the HIV service coverage achieved by all CBOs in the country. This ranking was made according to the denominator, based on numerical targets given to them by funders, and the numerator, which represented the actual number of people the CBOs reached on a monthly basis. In a worried tone he said "*their* denominator is 2000 but they are only reaching about 200 people a month." "Look," he showed me while pointing to their position in the diagram, "HOYMAS is at the very end! They are performing at the very bottom of all the [HIV-related] CBOs in Kenya. You need to talk to them about this." I then asked him how the denominator was calculated. He hesitated for a moment, then said "Well, this is the number they reported themselves. It is based on their funders' targets."

Next I spoke with the CBO director, John, about the matter. He mentioned that the government health officials came down hard on them about their "lagging performance." Then he responded by saying defiantly "Why do we have to report to them? This is a democracy! We do not have to report to the government on what we do—only to our funders!" He then continued, "Anyway, I don't understand how they come up with this number, the denominator." I suggested that we meet with the technical support unit representatives to further discuss this matter so that we have some clarity on how they calculate these rankings.

A few days later, John and his office manager met with the technical support unit director who began by mentioning the CBO's poor "national performance" in terms of coverage. John interjected and asked him to explain to all of us how one actually arrives at this denominator. The technical support unit director then went over to the flip chart in the corner of the boardroom and began scribbling down a series of numbers and calculations, explaining how denominators are, hypothetically, calculated for CBOs (see Fig. 5.1).

Although the diagram appeared as a jumble of numbers and calculations, the explanation seemed quite clear: all funders—be they the Impact Research and Development Organization (IRDO), the Centers for Disease Control and Prevention (CDC), the Elton John Foundation (EJ), the University of Manitoba (UoM), the Kenya AIDS NGOs Consortium (KANCO), the National Strategic Plan (NSP)—expected numerical targets to be reached. Some of these targets are overlapping, as a CBO might be expected to provide quite different services but to the same group of people—the denominator is not simply adding all the targets together, in other words. As the CBO director and his team began to understand the calculations, he and his office manager began to explain their agreement with another sex worker collective. On a monthly basis, they were expected to mobilize a large number of sex workers on their behalf. He also spoke about the referral work they conducted each day for one of the female sex worker CBOs in Nairobi. These activities, however, were not counted. It eventually became clear to the technical support unit member that there were a number of formal and informal arrangements between different CBOs, suggesting to him that the numerator was much higher than initially concluded by the technical support unit director. He quickly saw the error and then determined that the CBO should account for this added work in their numerator. He

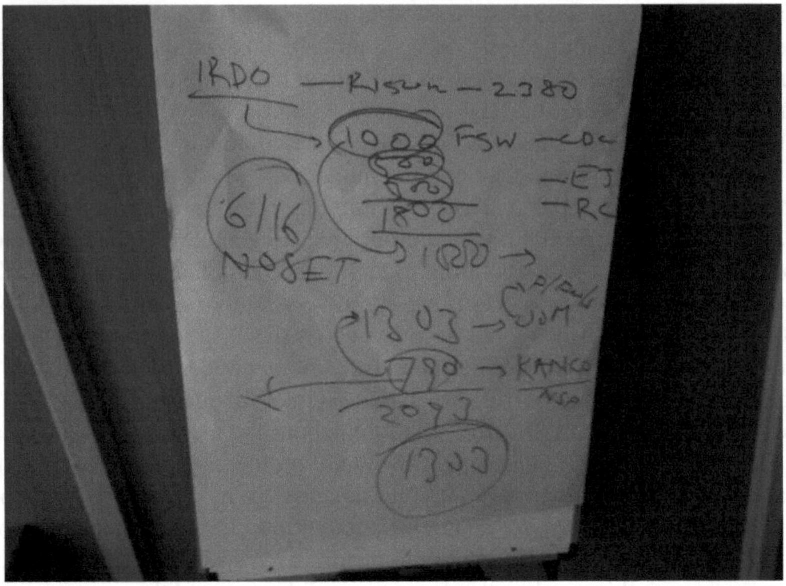

Fig. 5.1 Calculating CBO denominator to assess program coverage

also cut their denominator in half, realizing that it had not been calculated correctly to account for overlaps in services to the same people. Suddenly their performance ranking went up, considerably.

Noticing the unofficial work and responsibilities being shared between the different CBOs, I then asked the technical support unit member if it might make good sense to bring together representatives from the various CBOs to work through the mapping data to identify where their respective organizations were overlapping and where there were any coverage gaps or locations that were being missed. A US consultant, who also worked closely with the CBO, joined me in posing this possibility. Hearing the question, the technical support unit director smiled somewhat awkwardly saying "Oh, this cannot happen," and without offering any explanation, the meeting soon concluded. While the CBO staff seemed satisfied with the meeting, the consultant and I were left feeling puzzled by the lack of interest in actually working with CBOs to use the mapping data more effectively. I wondered: did the technical support unit representative view such a democratic exercise as undermining the regulatory influence they maintained over CBOs in Kenya? Such a process would, after all, involve the de-monopolization of evidence-based decision making. But the technical support member had also left out one vital piece of information from his elaborations pertaining to denominators. The various targets set by funders and given to CBOs were based on the mapping data shared with them by the Kenyan Ministry of Health, the technical support unit, and the World Bank. In other words, the mapping findings themselves exert a form of agency by enabling a consortium of transnational actors to govern the flows of funds to CBOs, while measuring their progress and ensuring their accountability.

Indeed the mode of power exercised by the technical support unit warrants critical examination. Its influence, I would argue, extends beyond mere neutral technical "support" to local Kenyan institutions in helping them realize their vision of improving health. Instead I would argue that the "technical support" model, a model that is increasingly promoted by large global health donors and multilaterals (although not without contestation), enacts a complex form of political governance that enables foreign academic institutions to influence HIV prevention "at a distance" (even when technical support unit representatives are located "on site"). Important for understanding the influence exerted by the technical support unit over local decision making arenas in Kenya, one must pay attention to how an international flow of funds ties in to its operations and how multiple affiliations are asserted through this rather ambiguous (but highly effective) entity.

The technical support unit in Nairobi simultaneously projects itself as a source of expertise, funding, and practical program implementation oversight, as it also directs local evidence generation activities (like "polling booth behavioral surveys"[6] and IBBAs) in collaboration with Kenyan government officials. The technical support unit receives funding from a Gates Foundation grant given to the University of Manitoba, which hires the members of the technical support unit, upon the approval of the Gates Foundation. The technical support unit officially represents the Gates Foundation when working in Kenya with the government health officials but they are also permitted to take a Government of Kenya affiliation when representing the interests of the Kenyan government outside of Kenya. For example, when the World Health Organization (WHO) and the United Nations Population Fund (UNFPA) held a global consultation in Ghana in May 2013 with member groups from the global Network of Sex Work Projects, the technical support unit representative based in Kenya took the affiliation of the University of Manitoba *and* the Government of Kenya at the consultation. Presenting multiple affiliations—something that sex worker activists also performed when asserting various memberships in different local, national, and global policy domains, depending on "the cause"—exemplifies and enacts a form of evidentiary sovereignty that is highly ambiguous and transposable. The interchangeability of affiliations (or the practise of layering them) positions particular entities and individuals in ways that maximize their decision-making influence across a number of spheres of expertise, and geographic scales and boundaries.

This form of sovereignty, it could be said, is rather tenuous, as the expected wielding of authority can also be challenged. This is what happened at the Ghana meeting when sex workers informally expressed their enragement toward the technical support unit member, who, as they put it was "not even a Kenyan citizen but is representing *our* government," thereby bringing the technical support unit representative's authority into question. However, with respect to the technical support unit's

---

[6] See for example Bhattacharjee, P., McClarty, L.M., Musyoki, H., Anthony, J., Kioko, J., Kaosa, S., Ogwang, B.E., Githuka, G., Sirengo, M., Birir, S. and Blanchard, J.F., 2015. Monitoring HIV Prevention Programme Outcomes among Key Populations in Kenya: Findings from a National Survey. PloS one, 10(8), p.e0137007.

influence within Kenya and its role in ranking CBO coverage—while holding the ear of government health officials and directing resources toward health system strengthening activities—it is exceedingly difficult for CBOs to challenge the technical support unit's influential role. CBO leaders were left wondering about the control exerted by the technical support unit over the flow of funds to them through the metrics they collate and share with the government officials and foreign donors. Furthermore, in addition to invoking multiple affiliations as a way to cast influence across various domains of policy and health service delivery, the technical support unit derives considerable influence in decision making arenas by virtue of their very role as technical experts—they hold and exert authority over the very definition and prioritization of "the problems" that "demand" intervention and require further funding. Important to note here is how such expertise directly aligns with the perspectives of the Canadian health scientists located at the University of Manitoba, where they draw their salaries.

5.3 Resisting Standards

In July 2013, as part of my responsibilities to the University of Manitoba I was tasked with providing technical leadership on an extensive qualitative research project, funded by the World Bank, through the University of Manitoba, but managed by the local technical support unit in Nairobi. The general objective of the project was to follow up on some of the findings from the quantitative mapping conducted the previous year; while the specific aim was to explore how the sex trade industry was organized and operated in Nairobi, across a variety of public venues that had been enumerated (see Lorway et al. n.d.).

The early meetings to develop and refine the protocol brought together Indian and Kenyan demographers, technical support unit representatives, health officials and members of the sex work community. As we discussed the protocol, there was some debate over having community researchers be trained to serve on the field team. One of the government officials said "We can't always trust the community," a statement quickly rebutted by the sex work leaders present at the meeting. In the end, the community won the debate to have sex workers serve as the field team. Then we all settled into our working group to review the protocol and re-worded the qualitative interview guides so that they would be understandable to the community and also addressed programmatic questions.

A few weeks later I began to work with the field team which was comprised of both male and female sex workers from HOYMAS and BHESP (Bar Hostess Empowerment & Support Programme), who both worked together under the umbrella of the Kenyan Sex Workers' Alliance (KESWA). The training served as a vivid window into the daily lives of the sex workers. Each day they would begin the morning by discussing the problems from the previous night they encountered at the hands of clients and police with respect to arrests, sexual violence and theft. As no health officials, technical support unit representatives, or clinicians attended the actual training sessions I delivered, the workshop participants grew more and more candid with me over the coming weeks. When it came time to purposively choose the hotspots where the workshop participants would conduct participant observation and qualitative interviews, we referred to an Excel spreadsheet list supplied to us by a Kenyan demographer who had worked on the previous nation-wide geographic mapping project. As we ran through the list of sex work hotspots together on the LCD projected image, there was plenty of chattering and murmuring, which eventually broke into open critiques of the information. The workshop participants insisted that a lot of the sites listed in the spreadsheet were either no longer active or the population size estimates were simply erroneous. One of the men who actually participated in the hotspot enumeration process as a field team member explained, "We were so rushed by the supervisors! You see, it wasn't really explained too well for the community, what the data was for, or how it was going to be used; so you see, Robert, some of the field team were just filling out the forms to get them finished!"

Without entirely discarding the list of hotspots, we continued to select the research sites, but drew heavily upon the sex workers' knowledge. Through ensuing discussions, our group realized that the hotspot-based female sex worker typology utilized during the mapping posed a problem for our qualitative aim of describing how the sex trade industry operated. Firstly, as the workshop participants explained, sex workers didn't necessarily stick to one type of hotspot. For instance, one participant explained, those who worked on the street, if they were unable to find a client that night, they would sometimes enter a nearby bar or nightclub to try to find a client; or they would contact their taxi driver by cell and head to a hotel; or they might possibly go to a sex den to find clients. In other words, instead of selecting separate, discrete hotspots, the group decided it was necessary for our qualitative study of the sex trade industry to actually group various hotspots together to form clusters of spaces or zones where sex workers moved about to conduct their business.[7]

Ultimately the study aimed to understand how the sex trade operated in Nairobi so as to understand the environmental risks they encountered. What we found instead were various security strategies that sex workers enacted, strategies that relied on various reciprocities between sex workers, waiters, bouncers and hotel security. As the following narratives illustrate, the sex trade was held together through a complex network of exchanges between multiple social actors. Furthermore, participants described their reliance on bar, nightclub, and hotel staff for physical and financial protection.

> [The bar staff] are the people who show us the people with money and those without. So they warn you when you are with [a potential client] who has no money, because they know everyone who comes to that club; those with money and those without. When you are spending time on a broke person, they tell you *nigutee masaa*, meaning you are wasting yourself. They are the same people who tell you that one is a policeman so be cautious and

[7] Interestingly, this paralleled how Ashodaya organized their outreach, grouping hotspots together into zones that reflected the flow of sex workers' movement between different types of spaces in Mysore.

> don't steal from him.... [The police officer] sometimes comes there pretending to be an ordinary guy ... they give us such information. (Westlands)

Bar and nightclub staff financially benefit from their relationship with sex workers by receiving a "percentage cut."

> The waiters and the small managers, they know the clients. Like when you go to [names a nightclub], you give them 100 or 200 shillings and they connect you to the clients. If the client is a foreigner or someone who is big, you pay 500 and they connect you to these people easily rather than you going to the men and asking them if they want sex. (Starehe)

'Beer' was a recurring theme in the participants' depictions of the exchange networks forming between sex workers, staff and clients. Holding these networks together was an "an economy of beer" that mediated the cooperative relationships between actors working in the sex trade.

> With the waiters, what you do is that after you have been given the drink, you send it back and tell the waiter to give you the money and you give him a cut from it. So that if the drink was 220 shillings you tell him to give you 150 and he can take the 70 on top. So if he returns like ten beers then he will have like 700 from you. (Embakasi)
>
> Yes of course you must go back to your pockets to give [the bar staff] something little. If you got 2000, you give them 200 and if you returned 4 bottles of beer, two are theirs and two yours. You must cooperate that way so that you continue benefitting from each other. (Starehe)

Such qualitative findings unsettle the reigning forms of quantitative evidence used to govern the response in Kenya, an epistemological leaning which tends to treat sex work as though it can be understood through the one-dimensional lens of behavioural and spatial risk typologies. Instead "sex work" in these narratives appeared as enmeshed in a complex field of social dynamics, underscored by power relations, transactions, and interdependencies. I raise this issue of the interconnectedness of social actors in the sex trade as an interpretive backdrop against which to consider a problem I pose next in relation to the planning of a clinical trial and the enrolment of sex workers, based upon the mapping data.

5.4 "We Mustn't Contaminate the Purity of the Control Arm!"

Although the uncomfortable marriage between Kenyan scientists and Indian program managers (arranged by a Canadian academic institution) led to a rather inflamed cohabitation, a more happy union occurred between the different technological approaches to monitoring health service delivery in sex worker populations. Through the South-to-South collaboration, the Avahan brand of enumerative technologies and the Kenyan bio-experimental techniques began to coalesce into an intervention regime that holds important implications for the power relationships between health scientists, program managers, health officials, and sex workers. Geographic mapping, for instance, was particularly appealing to the Kenyan health scientists because it not only offered a more systematic way to measure program coverage but it also created a sampling template with multiple layers of spatial and temporal randomization available for biological research. This became evident to me during the planning of a randomized control trial to test the efficacy of HIV self-testing technologies.

On a Friday afternoon in July 2014, I was asked to join a grant proposal for a randomized control trial to evaluate the efficacy of HIV oral self-testing kits among female sex workers. The application was to be submitted to the International Initiative for Impact Evaluation (3ie)—a granting agency funded by the Bill & Melinda Gates Foundation and UKaid through the UK Department for International Development and the William and Flora Hewlett Foundation. 3ie had selected Nairobi as a potential site for the randomized control trial, given the network of specialized clinics that served, simultaneously, as research and service delivery sites. I was asked to join the group, which consisted of a Kenya immunologist, a public health specialist based in Kenya, an Indian demographer, a Canadian infectious diseases doctor, and a Canadian mathematical modeler. I initially felt irritated for being invited at the final hour, an omission which speaks to how qualitative research is often valued in biomedical-oriented research—as an afterthought.

The mathematical modeller, in an effort to attend to the ethical dimensions of the trial, constructed the randomized control trial procedures along a step-wedge approach, which meant that the intervention technology (the self-testing kits) would be introduced incrementally to the population, as a staggered rollout, so that more female sex workers would have the advantage of accessing the technology over the life course of the trial. The team hoped I would be able to construct a qualitative study component around the trial that would follow up with participants, so as to help assess how the trial was proceeding, experientially. I agreed to join the project because I had been informed by a health official that the self-testing kits would be released to the Kenyan public within the next year or two and any information that could assess efficacy would be highly important to inform policy makers.

After reading the first draft of the grant, however, I felt uncomfortable with how the project intended to use the mapping data as a sampling frame to "randomly" select clusters of women at hotspots to be given the technology; while no technology would be given out at the control hotspots. The grant proposal also made no mention of consulting with local sex worker leaders on this project before it would begin. The proposal seemed to assume that these technologies could be randomly tested according to mapping data without social impediment. At a moment when our teams were trying to improve collaborative relationships with sex workers, drawing up memorandums of understandings around data sharing and ownership, I grew troubled that this oversight would undermine efforts to work more democratically with sex workers. I called for a meeting with two of the applicants, who I thought might be sympathetic to the ethical implications. I informed them that I was reluctant to continue to participate on this project as I felt deeply concerned over the uncollaborative nature of the trial. My ethical concerns overlapped with questions around the statistical sampling assumptions.

First I wondered about what harm could come to the sex workers if the trial proceeded without prior consultation with the community. Myriad scenarios of ethical problems sprang to mind, based on previous research I had conducted with sex workers in Nairobi and other parts of Africa and Asia. Here is one scenario that seemed plausible to me: a pimp or intimate partner might find the technology, force the worker to use it, and if she tested positive, she might be accused of infecting him. This could lead to situations of violence or the loss of her livelihood. Another scenario I imaged was as follows. Women might simply sell these technologies, given the major hit that sex work industry had taken in Kenya with the demise of the tourism industry due to highly publicized shootings and terrorist attacks. These technologies might quickly become mobile forms of capital in the informal economic sector, like ARVs already had in Kenya (Siringi 2004), which could circulate in unpredictable ways outside the confinement of the trial site. In a third scenario, women might give the testing kits to a friend or a fellow sex worker who may have had unprotected sex. What would happen if the women shared them with other people who would not necessarily be linked to the counselling services offered through the randomized control trial?

Related to the major ethical implications of leading a randomized control trial were questions pertaining to scientific integrity. Without carefully consulting with the communities who have the most at stake, the very notion that these "clusters" could be "randomly selected" was fraught with problems. As illustrated in the previous section, sex workers were indeed enmeshed in a complex web of social relationships, reciprocities and interdependencies, and thus while clusters of individual women might be "selected," the trial recruitment process would not necessarily be able to isolate these women's participation from the complex workings of their wider social networks. More simply put, I could imagine some of the women at one of the location merely texting their friends to join them at the hotspot where they were giving out the testing kits.

I suggested that these ethical-sampling complexities and other potential challenges for achieving "randomness" could begin to be addressed through a series of focus group discussions with sex workers or a very smaller pilot study conducted in close collaboration with community leaders. They would be best able to anticipate the ethical problems that could emerge in this randomized control trial. The two very sympathetic clinicians were appreciative of the issues I had raised and decided to back me up in notifying the concerns to the larger group. The other clinical scientists seemed somewhat receptive to the critique during the next Skype group call, but believed that these kinds of issues could be sorted out with a simple afternoon awareness session. The three of us who had previously discussed the matter, felt that the engagement with the community needed to be more extensive. I interjected, saying "You know, sex workers are now part of global networks, and if they feel we are not genuinely collaborating with them, they can easily have the randomized control trial shut down and bring negative media attention upon the trial." These words sealed the decision to include greater community engagement in the trial.

Our team presented a united front when we spoke to the impact evaluation specialist working for 3ie about the need to increase the budget to include a dedicated community engagement piece. When I expressed the need to consider a number of ethical issues and the need for community engagement, the 3ie specialist who was adjudicating the proposal reacted curtly by saying that this activity (informing the community) would "contaminate the purity of the control arm. We must not contaminate the purity of the control arm." I pressed on further by suggesting that if we fail to engage with the community the "natural" movement of sex workers between the sites might be greatly altered by the trial itself. I proposed that if we actually collaborated directly with the sex worker organization and they came to appreciate the importance of the study as a result, they might be more likely to go about their business, during the trial period, as they usually did. Then the 3 IE representative said "Well, we expect that your team will be able to manage the community anyway." Here the impact evaluation specialist made an interesting separation between the "science" of the randomized control trial and the management of the social dynamics, as though sociality stood outside of the randomized control trial as an external factor that could be merely controlled to ensure "unbiased" participant recruitments.

In the end, the trial did not go forward because of funding issues—that is, the reluctance of 3ie to accommodate community engagement as a dedicated component of the randomized control trial. Despite the failed grant application, this portrait of bio-experimental imaginings illustrates how the mapping data, in its visual depiction of order, seemingly ideal as a sampling frame for randomized control trials, inspires particular fantasies of decontextualized people, stripped of their social relatedness and complexity, and available to the interests of scientific bio-experimentalism.

References

Aiyar, S. (2015). *Indians in Kenya: The politics of diaspora* (Vol. 185). Cambridge, MA: Harvard University Press.

Booth, K. M. (2004). *Local women, global science: Fighting AIDS in Kenya.* Bloomington: Indiana University Press.

Dixon, V., Reza-Paul, S., D'Souza, F. M., O'Neil, J., O'Brien, N., & Lorway, R. (2012). Increasing access and ownership of clinical services at an HIV prevention project for sex workers in Mysore, India. *Global Public Health, 7*(7), 779–791.

Geissler, P. W. (2011). Parasite lost: Remembering modern times with Kenyan government medical scientists. In P. W. Geissler, C. Molyneux, & P. W. Geissler (Eds.), *Evidence, ethos and experiment: The anthropology and history of medical research in Africa* (pp. 297–332). New York/Oxford: Berghahn Books.

Krotz, L. (2012). *Piecing the puzzle: The genesis of AIDS research in Africa.* Winnipeg: University of Manitoba Press.

Lampland, M., & Star, S. L. (2009). *Standards and their stories: how quantifying, classifying, and formalizing practices shape everyday life.* Ithaca/New York: Cornell University Press.

Lorway, R., Lazarus, L., Chevrier, C., Khan, S., Musyoki, H.K., Mathenge, J., Macharia, P., Bhattacharjee, P., Isac, S., Kimani, J., Gaaki, G., Becker, M., Moses S., Blanchard J. (n.d.). *Confronting 'vulnerability' and 'risk': The everyday security strategies of female sex workers in Nairobi, Kenya.* Unpublished manuscript.

Sangaramoorthy, T., & Benton, A. (2012). Enumeration, identity, and health. *Medical Anthropology, 31*(4), 287–291.

Siringi, S. (2004). AIDS drugs being sold illegally on market stalls in Kenya. *Lancet, 363*(9406), 377.

Chapter 6
The Logic of Verification

Abstract This chapter portrays some of the less publically visible forms of activism waged in relation to the use of bio-experimental technologies to deliver routine health services to sex worker communities in Nairobi, Kenya. What becomes clear is how HIV surveillance techniques in Nairobi have begun to transform the very ground on which local sex workers conceive of and enact political resistance, a transformation that has produced a terrain of evidentiary politics: the new frontiers of political dissent surrounding the social effects of the highly graduated forms of tracking, measuring, and managing life, used in the name of HIV prevention and care. Evidentiary politics is certainly akin to biopolitics in the way that life and life processes are positioned at the centre of political contestation and inherent in the very technologies that seek to govern community participation. However, contestation centres on the means, instruments, and aesthetics of evidence production itself.

Keywords Biometrics • Clinical trials • Kenya • Men who have sex with men • Male sex workers • HIV

On September 18, 2009, 14 male sex workers living with HIV formed the organization Health Options for Young Men on HIV/AIDS and STIs (HOYMAS) by officially registering their collective as a CBO with the Kenya Ministry of Gender & Social Services. The collective started as a social support group with the aim of protecting their members from violence, providing care in times of sickness, and lending money in the event that one of them were running low on income. Initially members met in bars, pubs, and other places where they practised sex work. When I first met the founding members of HOYMAS in early 2010, they had begun to hold regular meetings in the board room of a sex worker clinic in Nairobi.

From the time of its inception, the group quickly began to fill a gap in health services, providing vital support and health information to their clients and peers. They were also instrumental in helping the Sex Workers Outreach Project (SWOP) clinic, run jointly by the Universities of Nairobi and Manitoba, to assemble a male sex worker cohort in 2009, a study which found exceptionally high HIV and STI prevalence (McKinnon et al. 2014). This cohort of more than 500 men was soon to form HOYMAS' membership base. In many ways the organization grew out of the HIV work they initiated in close collaboration with allied clinical scientists, coun-

R. Lorway, *AIDS Activism, Science and Community Across Three Continents*, Social Aspects of HIV 1, DOI 10.1007/978-3-319-42199-5_6

sellors, and government health officials that had long committed to working with sex workers.

In 2011, HOYMAS was officially launched as a CBO. The head of the Most at Risk Populations (MARPS) unit with the National STI/AIDS Control Programme (NASCOP), HelgarMusyoki, made a public address, during which time she imparted advice on safer sex and ARV adherence to more than 200 attendees. Also in attendance, UNAIDS representative Ruth Masha commended the group for forming the CBO, and according to journalist Dennis Nzioka

> [Masha] lauded the Kenya Government and NASCOP for their collaboration with MARPs groups that had helped expand the advocacy space that has enabled constituent members to be actively engaged in the national response. She cautioned the participants to be inclusive in their membership and open participation to not only MSM who are infected but to all as everyone is at risk and all are affected.

Representatives from the SWOP clinic such as the HIV prevention manager and a microbiologist, also attended the opening and extended a warm welcome to the community by inviting them to access free health services at SWOP. Of course this gesture was more symbolic. Most of the members in attendance for the event already participated in the cohort study running through the SWOP clinic.

Although the beginnings of the HOYMAS collective were very much rooted in sexual health campaigns and clinical service provision, the organization soon initiated a number of social justice initiatives that were more directly tied to civil liberties and global human rights. Among the events they organized included an international day against homophobia, biphobia and transphobia demonstration in 2011, which took the forms of a peaceful march to the Attorney General's office from Uhuru park; a flash dance near the Kenyan National archives; a screening of LGBTI documentaries at the Nairobi Railways club; and a public dialogue on homophobia themed *Mbona U Hate* (Why do you hate) at Nairobi City Hall. They also initiated a number of highly visible demonstrations in Nairobi, including a protest in front of the Nigerian High Commission in February 2014, with the aim of expressing their solidarity with LGBT Nigerians whose sexualities and genders were re-criminalized. Also in February, HOYMAS opened their doors to the asylum seekers who fled impending discrimination when the Ugandan tabloid newspaper known as the Red Pepper published the names and photos of a number of "gay Ugandans."

Staging visible protests only stirred the identity politics that were emerging in relation to international sanctions imposed on Uganda, giving rise to Kenyan parliamentary debates around the possibility of imposing more punitive ant-homosexual legislation. Responding to the idea of intensifying the criminalization of homosexuality in Kenya in March 2014, legislator Alois Lentoimaga said: "Can't we just be brave enough, seeing that we are a sovereign state, and outlaw gayism and lesbianism, the way Uganda has done?" Parliamentary debate culminated when the Republican Liberty Party submitted an Anti-Homosexuality Bill in the National Assembly, a bill proposing the public stoning to death of homosexuals. The author of the bill, Edward Onwong'a Nyakeriga, stated:

> The petition aims at providing a comprehensive and enhanced legislation to protect the cherished culture of the people of Kenya, legal, religious and traditional family values against the attempts of sexual rights activists seeking to impose their values of sexual promiscuity on the people of Kenya.
>
> There is need to protect children and youth who are vulnerable to sexual abuse and deviation as a result of cultural changes, uncensored information technology, parentless child developmental settings and increasing attempts by homosexuals to raise children in homosexual relationships through adoption, foster care or otherwise.

In response to this anti-homosexual rhetoric, HOYMAS and their allies, including local LGBT groups, local clinical scientists, health officials and program managers, decided to pull back from publically challenging the proposed bill and remained relatively silent, following the logic that posing no visible public opposition would eventually deflate the growing controversy, allowing the parliamentary debate to simply die out. And it did. This strategy aligns with Currier's (2012) discussion of how sexual minority rights organizations in South Africa and Namibia often enact "invisibility" during times of political hostility as an effective political strategy (Currier 2012).

The South-to-South community research project I helped to coordinate with male sex workers in Nairobi, took place amid this turbulent sea of politics—the influx of gay Ugandan asylum seekers, HOYMAS' public protests, and the growing parliamentary debates. When we began to explore the mental health issues facing male sex workers, the HOYMAS community research team composed the following question for the interview guide "how do you about feel about male sex workers fighting for their rights?" This question was interesting in that it offered a relatively indirect way to explore notions of stigma, but in a more politicized way. These were some of the responses we received from participants.

> Jeff: I think … [fighting for our rights] is something which is just. A right is something which you are entitled to and somebody cannot choke it away from you…. In this country *you have to go to the streets for your rights*, cause sometimes people know that these rights they are there but they still want to steal your rights.

> George: Okay, demonstrations are very good because they help us air out our problems, the things that face us in this world, the problems we face. Maybe *if you go in a certain street; like for us let's say Koinange Street is where we go at times. You go there… and we express all those emotions.* We are able to oppose even these bills that are usually passed in parliament; we go and say it is not fair to us and tell them we are normal people…. They are very nice demonstrations actually. Like let's say like 3 months ago there was a demonstration and people are like 'what are these guys demonstrating about?' and …we didn't care; we knew we were doing it for our lives, it would come to help us…. People knew what we wanted and you know … in the future we will be heard and they will let us have our freedom of what we want to do in the near future.

> Peter: Heh, those are the good people, and I am one of them.... When we demonstrate, the people from the media come, *we start from Koinange Street going all the way to Nairobi university way, going to Murang'a road, Ngara—we are known.* When that time comes, we usually do the demonstations so that Kenyans who are watching on TV can know that we are there, that there are male sex workers, gays…. Sex work, those men who have sex with men, so *they are here* in Kenya.

> Samuel: Being a male sex worker doesn't mean you are less human and … love is not a crime in any way. Loving a person, I don't know why it should bother you, loving a person,

or maybe, okay, I'm a human, whether I'm a male sex worker or whatever I do.... These people are the people, okay again they're the people who come for us, so at the end of the day, *I like whatever happens in the streets and I join it, and I scream a lot.*

Social theorists have long noted the crucial importance of public spaces such as "the streets" in the formation of political dissent, for visibly announcing defiance, with the goal of calling others to action. In this chapter, I want to describe some of the less publically visible forms of activism waged in relation to the use of bio-experimental technologies to deliver routine health services to sex worker communities. What I have begun to notice in Kenya is how HIV surveillance techniques have begun to transform the very ground on which local sex workers conceive of and enact political resistance, a transformation that has produced a terrain of evidentiary politics: the new frontiers of political dissent surrounding the social effects of the highly graduated forms of tracking, measuring, and managing life, used in the name of HIV prevention and care. Evidentiary politics is certainly akin to biopolitics in the way that life and life processes are positioned at the centre of political contestation and inherent in the very technologies that seek to govern community participation. However, contestation centres around the means, instruments, and aesthetics of evidence production itself.

For instance, in 2013 a controversy erupted surrounding the publication of a detailed map of sex worker hotspot in Nairobi by a group of African and US and Canadian health scientists. As a member on the email exchange list sent out to sex workers and their allies, I witnessed a frenzy of transnationally-circulating responses in the email thread, which seamed together global activist networks, academics, and civil society networks from across a number of African, Asian and North American countries, and beyond. In essence, objection to the publication of hotspots centred on the endangerment of sex workers, as such public exposure risked the intensification of police violence. The map not only enumerated sex worker "hotspots" in Nairobi, but geographically identified them with a specificity that allowed the reader to pinpoint the exact location of the venues, even though street names were removed. The sex workers I spoke to in Kenya who weighed in on this on-line protestation added that these scientists had no right to publish such information on their workplaces without their permission. Heated on-line protestation culminated in a response published in PloS One, the same journal in which the original article appeared. NGO directors, sex work community leaders, academics (including Carol Vance), and public health scientists authored the response and called for the outright removal of the map from the on-line, freely accessible publication. Part of the request for a retraction read:

We have read with interest the article "Enumeration of Sex Workers in the Central Business District of Nairobi, Kenya." We commend the authors on conducting much-needed research on sex workers in Africa, and the rigor of the research and methodology. We are however greatly troubled by the publication in the public domain of a map indicating sex worker 'hot spots' in Kenya, the location of which could be used by police and others to the violent detriment of the research participants involved....

Our experience working with sex workers across Africa and abroad, and in navigating the spaces where sex workers and police frequently meet, shows the intense vulnerability of this population to police brutality. This has been documented in Africa, and specifically in

> Kenya. Sex work is illegal in Kenya – a fact the authors themselves point out – which increases sex worker vulnerability to police violence and abuse of power….
>
> We would like to request that the authors and editors withdraw the map from the public domain with immediate effect. In addition, we would like to urge the authors to investigate whether any harm has been caused to the study participants in the area covered, and to implement measures to reduce potential harm in future.
>
> We would like to request the editor of PloS One to forward this letter of concern to the reviewers of the article and highlight their failure to notice the potential harm in the publication of such sensitive information. We recommend that PLoS One drafts an editorial policy on the additional scrutiny and caution required of publication of maps of highly stigmatised and marginalised populations, and include members of such groups in the review of articles in future.

Although the authors successfully forced the removal of the map, discontent among the global Network of Sex Worker Projects (NSWP) member groups continued to grow with respect to the use of geographic mapping techniques and enumerative practises. In 2015, the NSWP eventually commissioned a report in 2015 to express its views on mapping and enumeration, citing the example of Kenya as a cautionary tale.

> After the publication of the article and circulation of the [PLoS One] report, there was an increase of negative coverage of sex workers in mainstream media that included the secret and nonconsensual filming of sex workers at work. Security agencies conducted raids in some of the hotspots; sex workers and clients were arrested equally (NSWP 2015:8).

In another instance, negative public reaction sparked in relation to the leakage of the findings from a country-wide, World Bank-sponsored geographic mapping of "most at risk populations." Drawing upon the mapping findings, local government officials reported that Nyanza province, a popular tourist destination near Lake Victoria in the southwestern part of the country, "held the largest number of MSM [men who have sex with men] in the country" (Nzioka 2013). This public announcement was followed by three high profile attacks against individuals: one identified as a male sex worker, another as a gay man, and the third as a transgender woman. National and international news media characterized this brutality as the "local" reaction to the mapping study findings.[1,2]

> Several media houses mid this month reported that the National AIDS Control Council (NACC) had released figures purporting that Nyanza county had the highest number of 'homosexuals' compared to other regions sparking off debate. Another newspaper carried a report claiming that Coast was the region with the highest number of homosexuals. Religious leaders were roped into the debate that ensued with Muslim clerics arguing that NACC was promoting gay rights. Despite this furor, NACC came out to strongly oppose the article on the 'number of homosexuals' in the country saying they never released those figures. They further denied they were promoting homosexuality and clarified that they were focusing on HIV and that meant dealing with populations most at risk of HIV, mostly

[1] This story itself was circulated by Denis Nzioka, a popular Kenyan blogger and board of directors member of the male sex worker collective, whose posting was eventually carried by All Africa and ILGA.

[2] For further details of these attack see: http://www.nation.co.ke/counties/mombasa/Coast-gay-people-attacks/-/1954178/2888756/-/2e8f12/-/index.html

> men who have sex with men (MSM), sex workers and drug users. However, the reactions spilled over with the first reported cases of gay men and male sex workers being assaulted coming from Kisumu County in Nyanza.

HOYMAS, joining with their LGBT allied organizations in Kenya, including the Gay and Lesbian Coalition of Kenya (GALCK), and ISHTAR,[3] rose to defend the rights of LGBT people and condemned the attacks.[4] But the point I want to stress in these examples is how the knowledge generated by enumerative procedures—despite the seeming neutral and objective appearance of the numbers stirred particular postcolonial political anxieties and aggravated pre-existing political formations (such as those that cast homosexuality as an imported European cultural practise) as they "leaked" into the public domain.

6.1 Logic of Verification

> If there is no possible way to determine whether a statement is true then that statement has no meaning whatsoever. For the meaning of a statement is the method of its verification.
> —Karl Popper, *The Logic of Scientific Discovery (1934)*

The US and Canadian scientists I interacted in Kenya held great pride in the long-term relations of rapport they had cultivated with sex worker communities. Much effort had been made to include sex workers as participants in annual scientific meetings, for instance, where they were provided with free entrance fees. I witnessed staff buying food, tea and bread for sex workers when they visited the office, and their allied clinicians were quick and generous to respond to health crises in the community that arose when members were sick and had problems paying for or accessing health services offered at the specialized sex worker clinics. Indeed, most of the female and male sex workers I spoke with expressed immense gratitude toward the clinicians and the specialized services they offered to them.

However, with the new generation of surveillance technology, the imperative "to know the community" took an increasingly aggressive turn with the recent introduction of electronic fingerprint detection technology in the delivery of sexual health services to sex workers in Nairobi, Kenya (see Fig. 6.1).

In addition to raising human rights concerns in sex worker communities, the intentionality behind these biometric registration protocols exemplifies an intensification in evidence production processes that encircles what I call the logic of verification—an outgrowth of logical positivism that is sharpening monitoring and surveillance procedures to an almost juridical edge. By juridical, here, I am not merely referring to the similarity between biometric protocols and the use of

[3] The word ISHTAR comes from the name for the ancient Assyrian and Babylonian goddess of fertility, love, and war.

[4] The actual clinics were MSM receive in Kenya have also become highly politicized spaces. Between 2008 and 2015, there have been six violent attacks against men trying to access health services from one of the MARPS clinics.

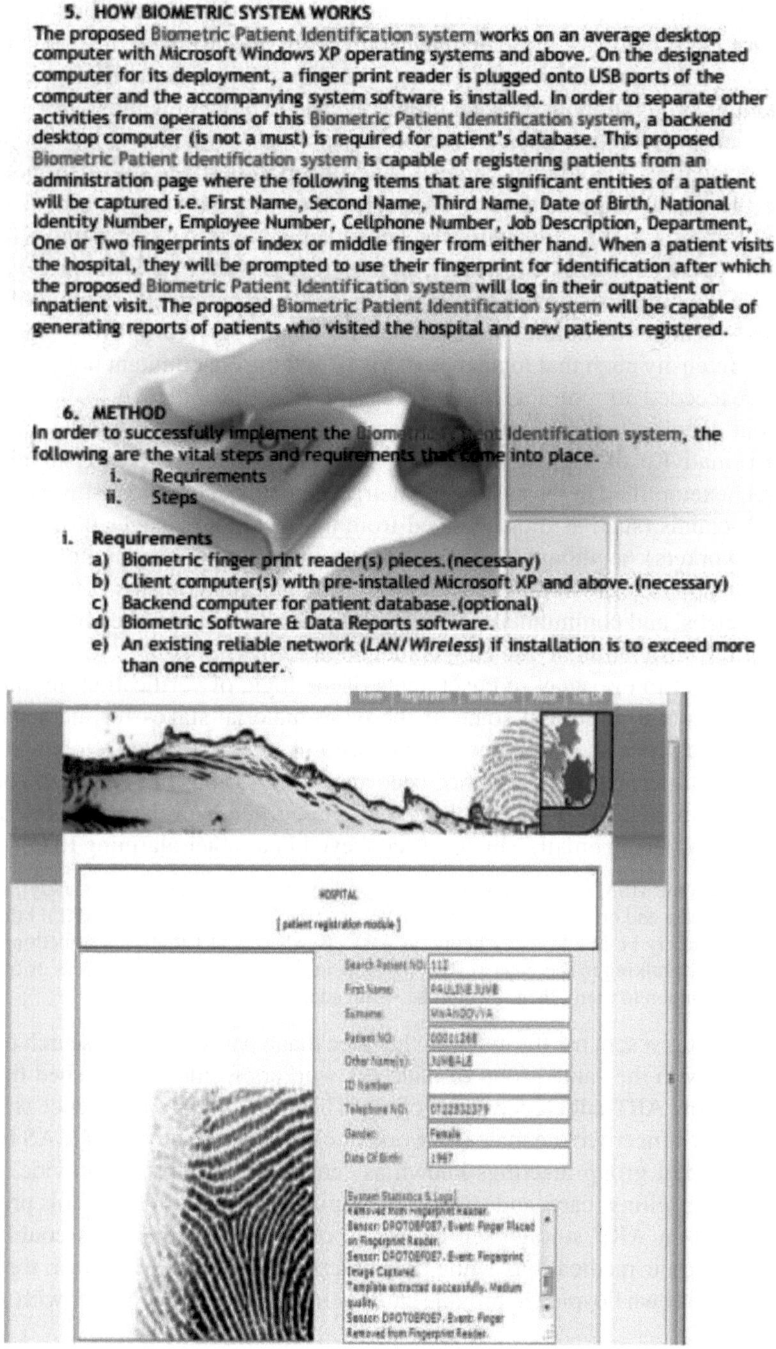

5. HOW BIOMETRIC SYSTEM WORKS

The proposed Biometric Patient Identification system works on an average desktop computer with Microsoft Windows XP operating systems and above. On the designated computer for its deployment, a finger print reader is plugged onto USB ports of the computer and the accompanying system software is installed. In order to separate other activities from operations of this Biometric Patient Identification system, a backend desktop computer (is not a must) is required for patient's database. This proposed Biometric Patient Identification system is capable of registering patients from an administration page where the following items that are significant entities of a patient will be captured i.e. First Name, Second Name, Third Name, Date of Birth, National Identity Number, Employee Number, Cellphone Number, Job Description, Department, One or Two fingerprints of index or middle finger from either hand. When a patient visits the hospital, they will be prompted to use their fingerprint for identification after which the proposed Biometric Patient Identification system will log in their outpatient or inpatient visit. The proposed Biometric Patient Identification system will be capable of generating reports of patients who visited the hospital and new patients registered.

6. METHOD

In order to successfully implement the Biometric Patient Identification system, the following are the vital steps and requirements that come into place.

i. Requirements
ii. Steps

i. Requirements

a) Biometric finger print reader(s) pieces.(necessary)
b) Client computer(s) with pre-installed Microsoft XP and above.(necessary)
c) Backend computer for patient database.(optional)
d) Biometric Software & Data Reports software.
e) An existing reliable network (*LAN/Wireless*) if installation is to exceed more than one computer.

Fig. 6.1 Electronic patient identification system used in Kenya: images and text created by Jomutech Agencies

biological information to verify truth claims in evidentiary legal proceedings (as in the case of DNA evidence presented in a court room, for instance). Instead, I attend more to the shift in relationships between clinicians, scientists, policy makers and communities brought about by such protocols, and explore how the logic of verification, in constituting a terrains of evidentiary politics, gives rise to new anxieties, ethical quandaries, ideological contests, and uncertainties. My aim here is not to suggest the literal implantation of Popperian logical positivism in global health practice; for certain, it is already firmly embedded in North American and UK public health epistemologies (McKinlay and Marceau 2000:27). Rather, I want to emphasize how the diffusion of this logic—from the experimental domain of clinical trials research to routine surveillance and health service delivery—gathered force and intensity such that logical positivism, and the concomitant notion of verification, exceeded its ontological moorings in scientific practice to become the prominent defining logic in the government of populations. As I will demonstrate, the performativity of logical positivism in routine monitoring and surveillance practices,[5] exemplified in the case of biometric protocols, moves to dismiss unverifiable truth claims (such as those derived from the local knowledges of community outreach workers), as though they furnish less important understandings for HIV epidemic responses. In so doing, it creates particular antagonisms between scientists, clinicians, and community outreach workers and other members of grassroots organizations responding to the HIV epidemic in Kenya.

With respect to everyday re-enactments of the logic of verification, let me provide an example to highlight some of the more material stakes for the scientists, clinicians, and sex workers I came to work with in Kenya. In late October, 2013, a conscientious microbiologist who had been analyzing various biological and behavioural data in a male sex worker cohort study based in a Nairobi sex worker clinic sent me the following email, which was conveyed in a rather alarming tone:

> I requested some MSM ART data from [the sex worker clinic running the cohort study]. The numbers in care and on therapy are extremely low (10 % of the HIV+ men on ART)! I think this could largely be due to many being on ART elsewhere, but I think it's something to consider when talking to the guys at HOYMAS. If instead it's due to poor access or other barriers (common to men), then it would be worth addressing.

The immunologist sent me the email in the hope that a participatory research project I had begun with the same group of male sex workers would help to shed light on the issue of low ART adherence at the clinic. The issue of ARV adherence was certainly of great concern to the male sex worker collective. Already HOYMAS had set up small support group meetings known as "encounter groups" to provide adherence peer counselling, care, and support to members living with HIV. This program also included an ARV storage service at the office so that members could more freely access their medications while they practised sex work. Moreover, the CBO had set up their own hospice to provide care for members who were sick with AIDS.

[5] My thinking around performativity (a term most commonly associated with the work of queer theorist Judith Butler), owes much to my conversions with S. Erickson and her intriguing work on the "performativity of statistics" (2012).

Alarmed with the clinic's news of low ARV adherence, two male sex work leaders and three community outreach workers formed a team and together we conducted consultations with 87 male participants (in groups of 6–8), over a 3-day period. Participants explained the following problems that related to low ARV adherence. Firstly the ARVs in the clinic were placed in a separate room from the other medications. Therefore, on entering "ARV room" one effectively disclosed one's HIV status before the other patients sitting in the waiting area. For this reason, many male sex workers had abandoned their ARV regimes and re-initiated their treatment at another clinic, funded by an entirely different donor. Secondly, a number of participants explained that they would sometimes bump into female friends of their wives or girlfriends at the sex worker clinic and therefore risked their own disclosure as gay and/or as a male sex worker. As a consequence, many male sex workers also shifted to another clinic, and to one that did not specifically cater to sex workers.

Together we shared this information with the clinic staff and appropriate changes were made to the storage and administration of the ARVs. The clinic manager also began to plan for the establishment of a separate clinic for the male sex workers (which has opened in April 2015). Although this consultation process took some time to complete, required funding, and was somewhat challenging to coordinate in a relatively short time period, the end result of this negotiated process contributed to relations of mutual trust between the CBO members, the clinicians, and the scientists, including the conscientious microbiologist. However, the discovery of ARV re-initiations at multiple clinics set off an alarm among clinicians and scientists managing the sex worker clinics, and soon justified the implementation of biometric protocols.

It is important to note that when biometric protocols are set up to detect co-enrolment between clinics across a given health system, clinicians are able to immediately "capture" and verify duplications in service utilization without ever having to wade into a consideration of the finer ambiguities of context. Therefore, with the introduction of biometric registration into routine service delivery, clinicians are able to control ARV access without the need to explore and understand the type of local knowledge that the conscientious microbiologist was interested in learning about from our participatory study and the community consultations. Furthermore, by immediately pinpointing service-use discrepancies, biometric protocols prompt individual patients (rather than organized collectives or community outreach workers) to provide personal justifications or even confessions, in the event that one is "caught" trying to subvert the system.

According to the HIV clinical researcher Jayajothi Moodley and her colleagues (2014), who are affiliated with the South African Medical Research Council, the employment of biometrics for the "real-time flagging" of people effectively avoids "co-enrolment," ensures "participant safety" and "data integrity" during clinical trials. However, a critical question remains: how will this experimental rationality operate in the more routine delivery, monitoring and administration of health services if biometric registration is rolled out as part of a larger intervention? In Kenya, HIV clinical services delivered to sex workers and sexual minorities are governed by a global mosaic of funders, influenced by the multitude of uneven public-private partnerships they mould. Thus, capturing duplications holds major implications for staking claims over populations and territories (or "catchment areas") in efforts to fulfil population coverage and biological targets negotiated with funders.

Couched in the ethical language of accountability to national and international donors, the logic of verification that underlies the push toward biometric registration marks an important shift in governing the HIV response in Kenya that speaks to the ideas of Vincanne Adams who argues that "global health," as a field of practice, has undergone a major epistemic transformation due to the influence of evidence-based medicine. Adams aptly characterizes this shift as involving a prioritization of experimental forms of knowledge (also see Nguyen 2010; Petryna 2009); increasingly, global health interventions are expected to meet the demands of randomized-control trial designs (Adams 2013). With respect to biometrics and HIV biomedical research in Kenya, these technologies have already been employed in clinical trials to detect co-enrolment (see for example: Mills 2011). More recently, however, biometric protocols have begun to be implemented in the HIV health service delivery sector. In September 2014, the government of Kenya called for the mandatory biometric registration of all people living with HIV enrolled in care. While this call is yet to be fully executed, currently the majority of specialized clinics catering to sex workers and men who have sex with men in Kenya are employing this technology for routine sexual health service delivery.

In the case of biometrics, I would argue that the logic of verification is fundamentally altering the relations between community outreach workers, clinicians and policy makers because these protocols enable clinicians and managers to by-pass the necessity of community engagement in HIV-related health service delivery. By setting up more juridical-like relations between clinicians and sex workers, the logic of verification simultaneously imparts and reinforces relations of distrust. Casting a shadow of doubt and suspicion over already stigmatized communities, this logic brings into question claims for increased funding, new programs, facilities and resources called for by sex worker-led organizations. In Kenya, it also inadvertently articulates with the wider criminalization of sex workers; for the force of the clinical demand for patient complicity with biometric protocols inadvertently colludes with the tenuous socio-political and legal status of those practising sex work, a group that is already highly restricted in their ability to demand equitable health services in state-sponsored health facilities. The introduction of biometrics has also given rise to begrudged reciprocities between outreach workers, sex work activists, and health scientists in Nairobi.

6.2 Protesting Biometrics

In July 2013 a small band of irate community outreach workers from the male sex work community, led by a local AIDS and sex work activist, held an organized protest at the entrance of an STI clinic in the commercial centre of Nairobi, the capital city of Kenya. The clinic, funded by the CDC/PEPFAR and managed by the University of Manitoba Medical Microbiology and the University of Nairobi, specifically catered to the sexual health needs of male and female sex workers. The group's enragement that day grew from the sudden introduction of fingerprint detection technology, deployed with the aim of registering and tracking the personal health information of sex workers. Their protest was loud, intense, but short-lived. It did not grab any front page news headlines like the other global human rights demonstrations they had led. But the organized dissent was highly effective in forcing staff to immediately concede to their demands; blocking the flow of potential patients (and biological samples) into the clinic prompted the clinic managers to halt the biometric registration protocol. Indeed the group were acutely aware of the clinician's vulnerability—that is, to retain funding, the clinic was required to fulfil monthly biological testing and treatment quotas to meet the targets prescribed by CDC/PEPFAR.

When I spoke to one of the activists following the incident, he exclaimed "They cannot disrespect the community like this!" and he mentioned that the NSWP would never stand for this "human rights violation." The symbolic irony of a "community friendly" clinic intending to fingerprint sex workers, many of whom were already regularly fingerprinted during periodic arrests by city police and *askaris*, certainly did not escape the activist; but it was the fact that the clinic managers had not consulted with the community on this protocol that had captured his anger, disappointment, and surprise. After all, the local and foreign clinical scientists who managed the clinic had had a long and well-established collaborative working relationship with sex workers since the immune quiescence studies (with HIV resistant sex workers) in the 1980s led by Allan Ronald and Frank Plummer (Booth 2004; Krotz 2012).

The clinic's attempted introduction of the biometric registration protocol was the first time this had been used as a routine part of service delivery to sex workers in Nairobi. However, it was not the first time that fingerprint detection technology had been employed in the HIV sector. In fact, biometric protocols have become common place in HIV-related clinical trials running at the Kenyan AIDS Vaccine Initiative (KAVI), based at Kenyatta hospital in Nairobi and Kangemi Health Centre, located 10 km from the city centre. Moreover, clinical trials scientists from KEMRI had already used similar biometrics to capture co-enrolment in three HIV prevention trials in Kisumu (Mills 2011). Following these trials, KEMRI scientists continued to use biometrics and electronic fingerprint detection as part of routine health service follow up in Kisumu and have extended it to Mombasa. And biometric protocols had been employed in Nairobi for a cross-sectional, bio-behavioural survey conducted with people who inject drugs in an effort to avoid duplicate recruitments in 2011 (personal correspondence with a senior KEMRI scientist).

More widely, Kenya has enlisted the aid of electronic fingerprinting technology during the March 2013 general elections to eliminate voter fraud. Although the technical infrastructure for the elections malfunctioned and resulted in majors delays in the voting process, this effort was part of Kenyan government's move to adopt e-identity systems for all citizens—an emerging trend promoted by multi-lateral development organizations (particularly the World Bank) in parts of Asia, Africa, and Latin America, under the guise that a shift to electronic identification systems would "grow a country's digital economy, and supports effective safety nets for disadvantaged and impoverished populations" (The World Bank 2014). In April 2014, the Kenyan government began the move toward biometric registration for all Kenyan citizens over the age of 12. Ushered in by the Uhuru regime, the system was implemented with the confidence that it would eliminate the mismanagement of social services funds, inhibit human trafficking, and thwart terrorism. In other words, the urgency to deploy biometric registration in Kenya's health systems joins the larger chorus on "anti-corruption" that echoes across the landscape of a number of African nations characterized as having "weak" or "failed" states. In September 2014, it became mandatory for all Kenyan civil servants to have their biometrics registered. This was implemented as part of austerity measures to eliminate the "wastage" of government resources perpetuated by "ghost workers." The outcome of this "purge" was that more than 12,500 people were not able to prove that they worked for the civil service (i.e., they could not provide appointment letters, education certificates, and or identifications cards).

The growing tensions and public contestation around the Kenyan government's larger adoption of biometric technology as a national citizenship verification tool set the stage for the unfolding of a biometrics controversy in December 2014, during an HIV technical working group meeting I attended in Nairobi. Organized by (NASCOP) and the National AIDS Control Council (NACC), the working group brought together a Kenyan born, North American-based senior epidemiologist who held close ties to Atlanta CDC; a regional UNAIDS representative; a ministry of health representatives from the HIV sector; a representative for a University of Manitoba-sponsored Technical Support Unit sponsored by the Gates Foundation, which sought to "transfer" the "lessons learned" from the India AIDS initiative known as Avahan to Kenya (see previous chapter); and two community outreach workers from HOYMAS along with their CBO director, who requested I join them to help deliver some of the preliminary qualitative findings from the participatory research project that we recently completed.

After the epidemiologist had guided the working group through a presentation that summarized the reams of accumulated data sources and bio-behavioural research findings that she had systematically gathered and organized, one of the NASCOP representatives, who manages the "MARPs (most at risk populations) portfolio" reminded the working group of the tremendous pressure she was under from the national Ministry of Health to implement biometric registration protocols at all the sex worker clinics under her jurisdiction. By January 2015 the government had planned to implement the biometric registration of all HIV positive patients in Homabay and Mombasa Counties and to expand the registration protocol to the remaining counties by March 2015. The NASCOP manager's concern was firmly supported by the UNAIDS representative and some of the other Ministry of Health representatives in attendance that day. Then the NASCOP manager asked the CBO director to respond to the issue of biometrics. The director's objections were threefold: (1) Sex workers were fearful of having their personal identities linked to the national electronic citizenship identification system, the development of which was well underway in the country; (2) given the criminalized status of sex work and sex between men, biometrics would likely inhibit their members from accessing services for fear of identity disclosure, and (3) because of what had recently happened in Uganda when computer hard-drives were seized from an LGBT NGO and the names of gay men were publicly released in the news media sex workers and MSM in Kenya did not feel that biometrics identity registers could be protected from public disclosure. Working group members were clearly moved by the CBO director's compelling arguments and eventually agreed with his position on the debate. Nevertheless they insisted that no compromise could be made for "injection drug users" receiving methadone—for biometrics were regarded as being essential to preventing them from harming themselves by accessing methadone from multiple clinics and thus exceeding the correct recommended dosage. No one from the injection drug using community was invited to the meeting to comment on this determination, I should add.

The MOH eventually decided to make biometrics "optional" for sex workers, but in CDC/PEPFAR-funded NGO-run clinics very few sex workers now refuse biometric registration across Kenya despite previous strong objections raised by community leaders and highly trusted outreach workers. The irony here is that the biomedical power to govern sex workers relies on the very structural vulnerability that it continually defines and aims to overcome with programs that enhance the treatment and care of sex workers living with HIV.

6.3 Experimental Market Logics

One morning in April 2015, a small meeting group assembled to explore the potential of a new research collaboration centring on the mental health needs of "African MSM." The objective of the meeting at first seemed quite straightforward. We intended to discuss how our teams could share and combine their respective research instruments, and data once it had been generated, so that a larger combined, cross-site data set could yield more compelling scientific evidence to call attention to this area of health. We hoped that the findings from the larger quantitative data set would influence future policy and funding priorities in the region. Twelve of us were seated at a long, banquet-style table in a somewhat shabby, overpriced hotel dining room in central Nairobi: two staff members from HOYMAS; two researchers from KEMRI (an clinical scientist and a social scientist); a clinical scientist affiliated with the University of Manitoba; a clinician who delivered services to MSM at KEMRI's clinic on a daily basis; and a "community mobilizer" (although "not an MSM", according to one of CBO members) who linked men who have sex with men to the KEMRI clinic. A representative from IAVI and a senior-level USAID representative were also in attendance that day, although KEMRI had invited them without the knowledge of HOYMAS or me.

A number of tensions lay just beneath the surface of the unfolding partnership that was developing between the meeting attendees. One year previously, HOYMAS had led a protest that had temporarily disrupted the operation of a KEMRI-run clinic serving MSM in another region of Kenya. HOYMAS members explained the circumstances behind the protest to me after the meeting. According to them, two men who have sex with men who had participated in an HIV prevention trial (and were required to drop out after testing HIV positive), developed major inflammation in their anal region. When they requested to be taken to the hospital for treatment and to have the cost covered by the KEMRI CDC-sponsored clinic, their request was denied. A wave of dissent grew until a community protest erupted against the clinic, an event which temporarily halted the clinic's operations. This protest did prompt KEMRI to provide the requested care to these individuals, and to change future policies.

The second tension related to the use of electronic fingerprint detection technology used to track patient records and service usage and to avoid co-enrolment during overlapping clinical trials (as discussed earlier in the chapter). HOYMAS adamantly re-declared its opposition to the use of this technology during the meeting. Yet, despite repeated refusals expressed by the members of HOYMAS, the KEMRI clinical scientist, anxious to use the technology for the mental health survey in Nairobi, persisted by saying "We can send someone to train your members at HOYMAS on how the technology works. We use it in [named a Kenyan city where KEMRI operates] and the community [there] doesn't have any problems with it." The University of Manitoba clinical scientist joined the KEMRI scientist by stating his concern that people taking the questionnaire might repeat it; for the questionnaire was being administered at two different sex worker clinics in Nairobi, including the one based at HOYMAS. "We will not be able to verify the participants without the biometrics," the scientist insisted. HOYMAS stood its ground on the issue and suggested an alternative, namely, that the questionnaire could simply be linked to the clinic registration I.D. numbers.

Thirdly, the HOYMAS staff members raised objections around the formation of an MSM research consortium that was established between KEMRI, the Universities of Washington and Manitoba, and IAVI. As they insisted, the consortium lacked any meaningful community representation. The HOYMAS staff members were also unclear as to the agenda and intent of this entity, which only seemed to include biomedical-oriented scientists.

Fourthly, our separate projects maintained different methodological commitments. Our participatory research program was framed by and centred on community interests, participation, and programmatic concerns. In addition to men who regularly accessed services from specialized clinics, we aimed to recruit and understand the mental health needs of men who did not access existing sexual health services. The KEMRI group, however, primarily was concerned with participants "currently in follow-up or enrolled in care." After we explained the broader intent of our project—to identify health service barriers and expand health service delivery efforts—the lead KEMRI scientist expressed his disapproval of our aim by adamantly saying, "Focusing on non-service users is an entirely different study." He reiterated that they only wanted to focus on MSM who were in follow-up.

Feeling perplexed, I wondered: Why were the KEMRI scientists so married to the focus on men who utilized health services? Why did they want to exclude the mental health issues of those who were *not* accessing services? Such an attention might point to access barriers that were important for early HIV detection and treatment and expand health services coverage. I also wondered why IAVI was interested in a project that seemed to have little to do with HIV vaccines. And why did a senior-level USAID official brave Nairobi's rush hour traffic to attend our small meeting on something as mundane as instrument development and data sharing? Despite the appearance of such a small group, the proposed research collaboration was expected to fulfil a larger ambition. Originally the lead KEMRI scientist said that "the larger sample size can help us to advocate for a greater recognition of the mental health struggles facing African men in same-sex relationships in the region." HOYMAS enthusiastically endorsed this strategic possibility and its potential to draw attention to the mental health needs of MSM in Africa. However, I eventually came to learn that the mental health survey masked another agenda that IAVI, KEMRI, and KAVI held—namely, to create a clinical trials population in Nairobi for future HIV prevention trials that IAVI would sponsor.

Although I was not a member of the MSM consortium, one of the clinical scientists copied me in on a long email trail that detailed the MSM consortium's projected activities over the coming year. The first communication in the email came from an IAVI representative in the USA who was attempting to plan out activities with KEMRI, their funding recipient, for the upcoming year. I summarize the lengthy correspondence and offer some analytic commentary below.

The **IAVI Representative** initiated the email dialogue by asking for an outline of the activities, budget and timeline for the upcoming year, so that additional funds could be earmarked. She then asked the consortium members for an update on the status of the mental health behavioural questionnaire, wondering if there were any activities that might follow on this project.

First Response Directing his comments to an Ivy League medical professor on the email group, a medical marketing expert, working for a private biotechnology company based in the USA, mentions a technology they were developing "that will be able to perform spot temperature measurements using a reader device close to the patient…." The marketing expert then asks the medical professor "Can you describe the *use case* as well as the *functional and performance requirements* please? It will help us determine if what we are planning will meet your needs" (emphasis added).

"Use case" is a term borrowed from software and systems engineering to refer to the patterns of interaction between a user and features of the software. Functional requirements refer to a set of technical details and processes that defines what a system is expected to do, which is captured in use cases. These terminologies are also applied in the field of health informatics to provide "a mechanism of describing the usage of a system … to identify big data usage patterns… commonly encountered in the health care domain" (Liyanage et al. 2014). The deployment of this lexicon is consonant with the emphasis placed on complex systems analysis in HIV implementation science (Schackman 2010).

Second Response The medical professor then refers the question of "the use case" and "functional and performance requirements" to the KEMRI scientist.

Third Response The KEMRI scientist, who agrees with the ideas presented in the first response, says

> We envisage that this [temperature detection device] [6] will be taken up by research participants currently in follow up (men who have sex with men, female and male sex workers). We would extensively brief participants about function (should be a colour change or other signal known to participant) that will prompt him/her to seek care at research clinic. Upon presentation, fever will be measured, and a blood sample subjected to an AHI [acute HIV infection] test algorithm, consisting of rapid ab [antibody] testing, and GeneXpert (when patients test negative or discordant). If the [temperature detection device] can transmit a signal that can be sent by a phone to alert researchers so that volunteer can be traced that will be ideal."

So in other words, the technology was expected to be useful in its ability to detect particular fevers that might be associated with acute HIV infection, and men using the proposed technology could be put on treatment as quickly as possible.[7] This follows the logic of "Treatment as Prevention (TasP),"or the idea that getting HIV positive people to take ARVs as soon as possible (regardless of their health status) will reduce HIV transmission at a population level (Montaner 2011). The KEMRI scientist continues:

> The device will be linked to the person – we would take biometrics (finger print scan, as we do already), this should first be tested in a pilot study. One important component is buy-in from the risk populations, specifically the MSM. I wondered if a student at [an Ivy League University] would have interest to visit us in Kenya and participate in the group discussions around this device. This can also be done by our team with consultation of the MSM/LGBT groups and sharing possible features of the device to be made. I would imagine that questions arise on whether the device will be cool… could potentially identify risk participants, and if they should [have it attached to them] at night as well during sex? Best would be a device that signals a body temperature of 38 ° C or higher.

Although the scientists make passing reference to the potential identification of an individual wearing such devices, the ethical concerns raised are primarily framed in

[6] I have deliberately anonymized a fuller description of the proposed technology so as to avoid disclosing the specific ideas of the consortium.

[7] Biomedical scientists maintain that the period in which an individual is most infectious is at the beginning of when they become infected, usually within the first six months. Fever (although a nonspecific symptom that can be confused for other illnesses such as malaria in places that lack appropriate diagnostic technologies) is considered one of the key clinical manifestations of acute HIV infection. (see for example: Cohen MS, Shaw GM, McMichael AJ, Haynes BF. Acute HIV-1 Infection. N Engl J Med 2011; 364:1943–1954 and Miller WC, Rosenberg NE, Rutstein SE, Powers KA. Role of acute and early HIV infection in the sexual transmission of HIV.CurrOpin HIV AIDS 2010; 5:277–282).

terms of community "buy-in" and whether or not MSM will find it "cool" and appealing to wear.

Fourth Response The medical marketing expert adds to the email trail by describing the proposed technology in greater detail:

> Our future product will be a [temperature detection device] and will send the temperature to an app on a phone continuously. This type of product can [be attached to the body] and be fairly inconspicuous. There are ... similar products about to hit the market from Temptraq, Stemp, and Feversmart. Click on the names to take you to their web page. There are watch-like devices that can measure temperature and one of them is called Basis Peak. You can check these out and I can reconnect in the future when our device is available.

Thus men who have sex with men, already considered as important global health research subjects, are also becoming envisioned as ideal marketing test subjects, with their participation implicated in the advancement of a family of technologies already marketed to consumers in the West. Below I present some of the images and text used to promote similar types of fever detection technologies by other companies (Fig. 6.2).

There is a rather jarring semiotic dissonance here between the depictions of the white babies carefully tended to with a ban-aid like health security device compared to KEMRI's proposed test subject—black adult male sex workers who daily face forms of sexual, physical, psychological violence and abuse. These kinds of devices are, however, the kind of celebrated "innovations" that now occupies a significant domain in the contemporary global health industry (Storeng 2014). It is highly unlikely that they will ever find a market in the impoverished neighbourhoods where most of male sex workers lived. Can this be seen as yet another example of Western scientists' attempts offshore clinical trials in low and middle income countries (Petryna 2009; Peterson et al. 2015)? What are the ethical implications of having Kenyan research subjects assume risks related to the disclosure of HIV status, sexual or work identity when these types of devices would likely find their market among higher income earners in the West?

Fifth Response The first KEMRI Scientist interjects again by referring to the high rate of seroconversion among MSM in a Nairobi-based clinic "Detecting AHI early and linking people to immediate ART could perhaps be a sub-study that we may want to develop in the consortium."

Sixth Response A second KEMRI scientist raises another other questions:

> Looks like it is still in development. There are clearly issues of accuracy, acceptability, durability and what the IRB [Institutional Ethics Review Board] might say. Also, what proportion of fevers will be attributable to early HIV infection? And how scalable is this? Good for a study, but how would it work on a community/population level, or is that not a consideration and *it would be used only in studies*? [Emphasis added]

Beyond questions of how to navigate ethical hurdles and the specificity of fevers to HIV infection, there is a layering of experimental logics in this response. The KEMRI scientist suggests that the technology might prove useful as a tool for future

Temptraq

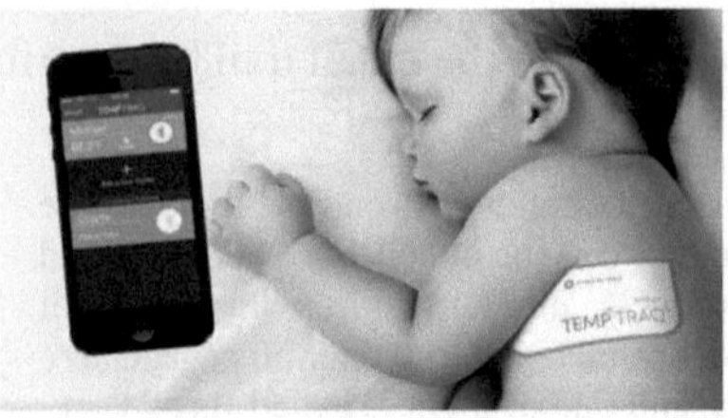

Promotional text accompanying this image: "This feels like the future of health technology. This is the temptraq and it is like a band-aid, except is it's a thermometer. Meant to monitor a baby with a fever over a 24 hour period, the adhesive strip contains a thermometer, a flexible battery, and blue tooth. Press the start button, apply it to the skin and it pairs with the phone to give you continuous temperature information the app also allows you to monitor the temperature of multiple strips in case you have multiple children. And you get an alert if the temperature reaches a particular threshold. You can take notes about when drugs were taken and even send charts to a doctor."

STEMP

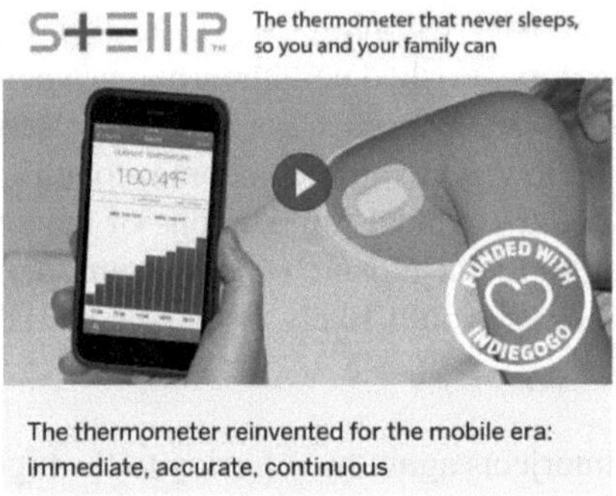

Fever Smart

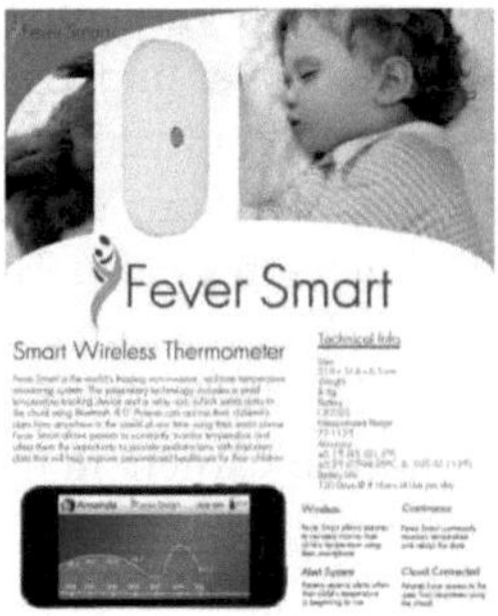

Fig. 6.2 Temperature detection advertisements

experiments, even if the device cannot be used in public health programs to accurately determine whether or not fevers are attributed to acute HIV infection. Therefore, value is perceived in having men who have sex with men participate in the testing of the temperature detection device not because it holds direct benefit to the community, but because their participation could generate a resource to further the experimental enterprise itself.

The second KEMRI scientist continues:

> If the device were far enough along, we could try a small pilot at each of the three sites. It sounds like all three sites will be doing fingerprinting, is that correct? We need to set up a

> system of trading the digital info periodically (biweekly? monthly?) to be able to detect participants who access services or try to enrol across sites, and we need someone to take the lead on setting that up and then analysing the data. Maybe a student? Even a student would need a little money.
>
> I still love the idea of looking at HIV strains/genotypes across the three sites. Ideally, it would include MSM, heterosexual men, FSW and lower risk females across the three sites, but we could start just by looking at samples from MSM to assess similarities and differences in HIV strains. We can't get enough money to do a full study, but could we do a pilot that could then serve as the basis for a larger proposal? … [N]ot sure if this is of interest to IAVI, but should be of interest to the MOH, and isn't the IAVI money from USAID in part to support the Kenyan MOH?

Responses throughout the email trail illuminate the techno-scientist utopias of mastery and efficiency (biometric tracking to avoid co-enrolment, the swift transfers of digital information, and genotypes to reveal transmission patterns at the molecular level) that animates the bio-experimental regime. It is also worthwhile noting the recurring reference made to "students," which is telling of how scientific labour in experimental enterprises is organized. And the flows of funding from USAID, to IAVI, to KEMRI—with its linkage to the Kenyan State, importantly, suggests how a Kenyan government unit may become entangled in US commercial and scientific enterprise.

After reading and re-reading the entire correspondence, I was still left feeling puzzled: how did this conversation relate back to the mental health study, as originally posed by the IAVI representative? A few days later, the first KEMRI scientist followed up on the email trail by responding.

> The primary idea is to assess mental health challenges, stigma, substance use, etc., in MSM who are accessing care (defined as men who are in follow up)…. We reasoned that as we are working towards building a potential HIV prevention trial population assessing challenges in men who are enrolled in care is of primary interest.

This response helped make clear that the findings for the mental health questionnaire primarily were also intended to serve the interest of assessing how well "the MSM community" would be able to participate in future HIV prevention trials sponsored by IAVI. While our participatory study included MSM who did not access services, to shed light on health service utilization barriers, the KEMRI mental health studies aimed to build a clinical trial population from a pool of already "compliant" health service users—therefore excluding a consideration of how to expand services to those who may be the harder to reach. Following this experimental logic, members of the MSM consortium eventually decided to undertake a Simulated Vaccine Efficacy Trial (known as SiVET in the clinical science literature) among male sex workers in Nairobi. This involved administering an already approved hepatitis B vaccine that required 3 separate doses to test how well the male sex workers could adhere to a hypothetical vaccine trial.

The larger point that can be drawn out here is how the circulation of logics, technologies, and procedures between experimental and routine health service domains creates a blurring in boundaries for service users such that it becomes increasingly difficult for sex workers to know when they are accessing regular health services or participating in medical research. Indeed clinics for "key populations" funded by CDC/PEPFAR (and not only in Kenya) are already firmly entrenched in bio-experimentalism through ongoing cohort studies, and immunological and biological assessments.

6.4 Trial Acceptability

Johanna Crane (2013) described the rapid expansion of an HIV research program and industry in Uganda as it began in the 2000s, shifting with the changes in ARV delivery systems and the convergence of international medical research agendas. International involvement in medical research in Kenya, however, follows a longer historical trajectory when the establishment of KEMRI in the 1970s, in collaboration with its transnational partners, began to draw control away from the Kenyan government and local academic institutions (Geissler 2011). In the 1980s, the fortuitous meeting of University of Manitoba microbiologist Allan Ronald with the University of Nairobi head of the Microbiology Department, Herbert Nsanze, gave rise to a scientific partnership between the Kenyan and Canadian universities. The partnership formed around the study and treatment of an outbreak of cancroid, a genital ulcerative disease, among female sex workers living in an impoverished neighbourhood in Nairobi. The collaboration gave birth to the Majengo Observational Cohort Study (MOCS) in 1984, which is now considered one of the world's longest running observation cohorts (Bandewar et al. 2010). In the late 1980s, with the discovery of HIV resistance among a small sub-group of this cohort, this research collaboration became a major player in the international HIV scientific knowledge production field. This position was further reinforced with subsequent clinical research accomplishments including the renowned male circumcision randomized control trial led by Robert Bailey of KEMRI and Stephen Moses at the University of Manitoba (Bailey et al. 2007; Krotz 2012) and a skilled team of University of Nairobi microbiologists, including the late Jeconiah Oliver Ndinya-Achola (Krotz 2012).

Despite the positive contributions and accumulated accolades, including a mention in *Time* magazine,[8] this partnership also came under public scrutiny. On January 2007, journalist Stephanie Nolan published an article entitled "Sex Slaves for Science?" in the Canadian National Newspaper known as *The Global and Mail*. Nolan raised critical questions around the long-term involvement of sex workers in the cohort and their continued poverty, thus directing ethical queries toward a number of Canadian and Kenya scientists who established prominent careers on the long standing MOCS. Nolan quotes one of the women who had been a long-time participant in the MOCS and some of the clinic staff in her article.

[8] The male circumcision trial results were list as one of the 10 top medical achievements of 2007 by Time magazine. [http://www.theglobeandmail.com/life/canadian-researcher-honoured-by-time/article1092165/]

'I feel they taken advantage of me, because I've made such a big name all over the world [for the project] but I'm still in this business. I need something to lift me out of Majengo.'

Her frustration is echoed by the Kenyan nurses and counsellors at the little clinic. 'These women, 20 years later, they're still in these small rooms,' one irate staffer says, adding that she and her colleagues suspect the researchers privately want the women to keep working: 'With no sex workers, what would happen to their research?'

According to Prof. Ngugi, who has worked intimately with the women for 20 years, 'this has given the world such a huge body of knowledge, but what has the world done to help them change? … Quite clearly there is an imbalance.'

During the South-to-South community research project I conducted with male sex workers in Nairobi, some of the participants also raised objections to clinical trials. A 21-year-old male sex worker, for instance, characterized clinical trials as not meeting the interests of local communities.

People are coming from outside the country. They start these researches and whenever they are done with these researches they never release the results to the community. So people don't know what they were researching on, what they found out, how they are going to deal with the problems they found out and they feel like they have been neglected, they feel like they have been used because this people are not aware of how these researches are helping them because you can't come in and get information from me and you don't tell me how it is going to help me in any way and you just leave. That is not right.

One theme running across a number of the transcripts was the notion that research subjects were treated similarly to "guinea pigs."

I have issues, I don't know. I have issues with the whole idea of it's a research, I have fears from the movies I have watched, the guinea pigs or lab rats. I have issues, because I am not sure. I don't like the whole idea of a person observing me trying to see how I react. I like something that has been approved, so the whole idea of … No I have issues … I have a lot of issues. [23 years old]

Prior to the South-to-South community research project, I led a 3-year HIV vaccine acceptability study, between 2010 and 2013, in collaboration with leaders and activists from communities of make sex workers and men whom have sex with men in the urban centres of Kisumu, Nairobi, and Mombasa. Some of the research participants mentioned their specific concerns regarding HIV vaccine trials. The objections were primarily raised at the Nairobi site where KAVI ran most of its HIV vaccine and other prevention trials.

Collin: I think [HIV vaccines] should be tested universal[ly], not direct to one community alone…I have seen they are coming too much to the MSM community. So, I would prefer a little change so that it would be universal. [Nairobi, 24 years old]

David: What is there for the MSMs? Are they going to be pioneers of this thing or are they just going to be those people were used along the way to get what we wanted? How well is their health taken care of thereafter? [Nairobi, 22 years old]

Interestingly, however, the majority of participants across the three urban sites expressed enthusiasm when asked if they would be willing to participate in future HIV vaccine testing.

Abasi: I would love very much (to participate) because I know that it is going to help the sex workers and the gay community to be more healthy and not be sick; who wouldn't want to participate in such a thing. [Kisumu, 28 years old]

Baraka: I would be willing to participate in order to lower the rate of infection or transmission or re-infection of HIV and AIDS in the community and also globally. [Kisumu, 27 years old]

Chilemba: I would like to participate … because when I benefit even my fellow and the community will benefit, not only for the MSM. [Mombasa, 23 years old]

Ben: I would participate for the betterment of myself and my fellow MSMs or rather the fellow Kenyans at large. [Mombasa, 26 years old]

Hali: I would do that [get involved in clinical trials] because sometimes it is important to be part of a good course. Because for us, for instance, to ascertain a certain medicine is working of course we have to try it on human beings regardless of how many other animals that we have used. It is always important to be involved in such kind of a thing, yeah. [Nairobi, 27 years old]

Hamadi: Yes … because I will help the family, the society, the neighbours, anybody who will come across it. [Nairobi, 24 years old]

Benard: Actually I would participate in order to support my MSM community so that I would support my MSM community and the nation at large; you know when you participate you are patriotic to your country. [Nairobi, 34 years old]

Despite the numerous altruistic and nationalistic declarations of "willingness to participate," the majority of participants interviewed in the HIV vaccine acceptability study made a number of recommendations directed at the clinical trials specialists. Based on their own experiences, one of the main areas in which they hoped for improvement related to transparency (also see Doshi et al. n.d.).

Geoffrey: They need to inform the MSM community on how and when to do the research and the benefit of the research to the MSM community…. They [the MSM community] should be informed about the results and the researchers should keep their confidentiality and also inform them what is next in the MSM community. [Kisumu, 20 years old]

Hanif: They should explain to them what research is about not enrolling someone into research because he is an MSM. He [the participant] keeps hearing there is a research that is starting, that there is money—one thousand or two, three thousand—he will run for the money … because it is someone's life you have to be sure of what is going on…. You run for the better option because research comes in every type and researchers are everywhere in town. [Mombasa, 20 years old]

Mark: They ought to train [the MSM community] more about the research and why they are making them take the vaccine. [Nairobi, 24 years old]

The second area where they made recommendations related to how clinical trial staff should establish rapport with them, suggesting that they should involve the community more directly in the running of the research trial itself:

Jamal: They should use the MSM during the research; they [should] create employment for this MSM, using them as a tool for the research, so they should involve them, at least; they became field officers. [Kisumu, 19 year old]

Brian: They need to create that rapport; they need to give feedback constantly whether it is negative or positive…. They should not spoil [the relationship] by just cutting the link all of

> a sudden [when the trial is complete] … it creates an impression where people feel they were just used; they are guinea pigs. [Nairobi, 32 years old]

Many of the participants were also adamant that trial scientists need to ensure the proper dissemination of the results at the conclusion of the clinical trial:

> Paul: They should tell [the MSM community] on the result and in fact talk to them well and explain to them what the research has come out. [Kisumu, 21 years old]

> Kito: They are supposed to return the feedback … you will ask yourself, these people have taken our blood … these people keep on testing us … what have they found it's okay or it's not okay?… We need some feedback of course of which I don't see mostly in many researchers. [Mombasa, 20 years old]

> Vincent: Well for those who participated in the research, they should be given the treatment for free and they should be informed more on … whatever that will be discovered or not that because like in the researches that we have had before or I have heard of people never get the feedback afterwards; they are just told thank you we are through with the project. [Nairobi, 26 years old]

In recent years, in adherence to global guidelines, the Kenyan AIDS Vaccine Initiative, which was founded in 1998 and had completed eight HIV vaccine trials by 2013, began to prioritize community engagement by setting up community steering committee with the intention of increasing community literacy and acceptability, following their receipt of a 1.8 million dollar Canadian HIV Vaccine Initiative (CHVI) grant. Some of the sex worker activists and other community leaders involved in HIV vaccine acceptability study, after meeting with the trial scientists in 2014 and 2015, have come to take an active role in educating the KAVI trial staff on the ethical concerns that are peculiar to sex workers.

6.5 Affecting Science

In November 2014, as the community research team of male sex workers began to analyse their sexual life history interviews, the conscientious microbiologist (who you may recall from earlier in this chapter) asked to meet with me to discuss some of the biological research their team planned to conduct with the male sex worker cohort they assembled at the sex worker clinic in Nairobi. He discussed a new approach for anal mucosal sampling for understanding the infectivity of the HIV via anal sex. This technique built on previous mucosal sampling techniques used by the University of Manitoba team to explore immune quiescence (Schellenberg and Plummer 2012). He was concerned that the sampling methods, although important for scientific exploration, might not be well-received by the men, "You know you have to wash the anal region with saline before you can actually take the sample. I am worried that this is too invasive for the guys." I responded by saying "Why don't you explain this issue to the community researchers and ask them directly. Can you try to explain some of the science behind it?" I suggested. This was, perhaps, a rather provocative request, expecting the lab scientist to "leave the lab," so to speak, and enter the messier realm of social analysis. But he happily agreed.

The next day, he met with the community researchers in small groups of four and five individuals, while the others practised analysing their qualitative interview transcripts based on analytic techniques I had taught them. The microbiologist showed the small groups a simplified PowerPoint presentation that outlined the scientific contributions that his team hoped to make with the anal mucosal samples, and explained how this would help reveal the role mucosal cells played in HIV acquisition. Then he detailed the actual biological sampling procedure. He was surprised by the enthusiasm of the groups who did not think that the procedure was too invasive for a number of reasons. Firstly many of their community members had already participated in a previous study led by the University of Nairobi that screened for STIs in the anal and genital region. This was a positive experience for the community because of how the study staff interacted with them and treated their infections. More generally they explained that the community was fine with the anal examinations. Male sex workers commonly felt as though they were not as thoroughly examined as female sex workers.[9] While the women received regular speculum exams, the men were rarely given anoscopy (anal speculum) examinations during regular health check-up at sex worker clinics, they claimed. Thirdly the young men expressed great interest in the science itself, and how this new information might help explain their extreme HIV vulnerability.

The kinds of interactions I observed that day helps to reveal how the mutual affecting of scientists and communities somehow alters the very rhythms of scientific production practises, perhaps slowing it down, but also opening up new lines of questions that connect abstract universalistic procedures to the grounded life history of clinical research in Kenya. Indeed "HIV scientific knowledge" produced in Kenya over the years does not merely exist as a linear accumulation of successive findings, even though it is sometimes articulated by scientists in these terms. HIV scientific advancements or "progress" instead proceeds within an irregular, heterogeneous and highly contestable field of social practises and shifting social networks.

References

Adams, V. (2013). Evidence-based global public health. In J. Biehl & A. Petryna (Eds.), *When people come first* (pp. 54–90). Princeton: Princeton University Press.

Bailey, R. C., Moses, S., Parker, C. B., Agot, K., Maclean, I., Krieger, J. N., Williams, C. F., Campbell, R. T., & Ndinya-Achola, J. O. (2007). Male circumcision for HIV prevention in young men in Kisumu, Kenya: A randomised controlled trial. *The Lancet, 369*(9562), 643–656.

Bandewar Sunita, V. S., Joshua, K., & JamesV, L. (2010). The origins of a research community in the Majengo observational cohort study, Nairobi, Kenya. *BMC Public Health, 10*(1), 630.

Booth, K. M. (2004). *Local women, global science: Fighting AIDS in Kenya*. Bloomington: Indiana University Press.

[9] This was consistent with the feedback from the community consultation with 87 male sex workers I had coordinated with HOYMAS.

Crane, J. T. (2013). *Scrambling for Africa: AIDS, expertise, and the rise of American global health science*. Ithaca: Cornell University Press.

Currier, A. (2012). *Out in Africa: LGBT Organizing in Namibia and South Africa*. Minneapolis: University of Minnesota Press.

Doshi, M., Avery, L., Kaddu, R. P., Gichuhi, M., Gakii, M., du Plessis, E., Dutta, S., Khan, S., Kimani, J., Blanchard, J., & Lorway, R. (n.d.). *Rethinking willingness to participate: Historically grounded recommendations for engagement, recruitment & enrolment of Kenyan MSM in future HIV prevention trials*. Unpublished manuscript.

Erikson, S. L. (2012). Global health business: The production and performativity of statistics in Sierra Leone and Germany. *Medical Anthropology, 31*(4), 367–384.

Geissler, P. W. (2011). Parasite lost: Remembering modern times with Kenyan government medical scientists. In P. W. Geissler, C. Molyneux, & P. W. Geissler (Eds.), *Evidence, ethos and experiment: The anthropology and history of medical research in Africa* (pp. 297–332). New York/Oxford: Berghahn Books.

Global Network of Sex Work Projects (NSWP). (2015). *Mapping and population size estimates of sex workers: Proceed with extreme caution*. http://www.nswp.org/tags/ethical-research.

Krotz, L. (2012). *Piecing the puzzle: The genesis of AIDS research in Africa*. Winnipeg: University of Manitoba Press.

Liyanage, H., de Lusignan, S., Liaw, S. T., Kuziemsky, C., Mold, F., Krause, P., Fleming, D., & Jones, S. (2014). Big data usage patterns in the health care domain: A use case driven approach applied to the assessment of vaccination benefits and risks: Contribution of the IMIA primary healthcare working group. *Yearbook of Medical Informatics, 9*(1), 27.

McKinlay, J. B., & Marceau, L. D. (2000). To boldly go. *American Journal of Public Health, 90*(1), 25–33.

McKinnon, L. R., Gakii, G., Juno, J. A., Izulla, P., Munyao, J., Ireri, N., ... & Musyoki, H. (2014). High HIV risk in a cohort of male sex workers from Nairobi, Kenya. *Sexually Transmitted Infections*, *90*(3), 237.

Mills, L. (2011). *Preventing clinical trials co-enrollment through biometric participant identification: The experience of three HIV prevention trials in Nyanza Province* (Lisa Mills – CDC / KEMRI). Presentation delivered at The Annual Review Meeting (Monday, January 17, 2011). University Of Nairobi Std/Aids Collaborative Group, Mayfair Court Southern Sun, Nairobi. http://www.ajhsjournal.or.ke/?p=1284

Montaner, J. S. (2011). Treatment as prevention—A double hat-trick. *The Lancet, 378*(9787), 208–209.

Moodley, J., Govender, V., Naidoo, S., Govender, D., Ramjee, G., & Charls, P. (2014). Ethical considerations in implementing a biometric co-enrolment prevention system in clinical trials in South Africa. *AIDS Research and Human Retroviruses, 30*(S1), A202–A202.

Nguyen, V. K. (2010). *The republic of therapy: Triage and sovereignty in West Africa's time of AIDS*. Durham: Duke University Press.

Nzioka, D. (2013). *Attacks on LGBTI, sex workers sorrying*. http://ilga.org/attacks-on-lgbti-sex-workers-worrying/.

Peterson, K., Folayan, M. O., Chigwedere, E., & Nthete, E. (2015). Saying 'No' to PrEP research in Malawi: What constitutes 'failure' in offshored HIV prevention research? *Anthropology & Medicine*, *22*(3), 1–17.

Petryna, A. (2009). *When experiments travel: Clinical trials and the global search for human subjects*. Princeton: Princeton University Press.

Schackman, B. R. (2010). Implementation science for the prevention and treatment of HIV/AIDS. *Journal of Acquired Immune Deficiency Syndromes* (1999), *55*(Suppl 1), S27.

Schellenberg, J. J., & Plummer, F. A. (2012). The microbiological context of HIV resistance: vaginal microbiota and mucosal inflammation at the viral point of entry. *International Journal of Inflammation, 2012*, 1–10.

Storeng, K. T. (2014). The GAVI Alliance and the 'Gates approach' to health system strengthening. *Global Public Health, 9*(8), 865–879.

World Bank. (2014, June). *Digital identity toolkit: A guide for stakeholders in Africa*. http://www-wds.worldbank.org/external/default/WDSContentServer/WDSP/IB/2014/10/08/000456286_20141008100737/Rendered/PDF/912490WP0Digit00Box385330B00PUBLIC0.pdf.

Conclusion

It is important to pause occasionally to think about what moves and shakes the world of HIV activism and science in terms of significant events: grand announcements of scientific breakthroughs, international headline-grabbing demonstrations, or stunning political rhetoric that declares new policy directions. Indeed we inhabit a moment in which scientific and technical advancements conjure compelling visions of "success" against the HIV epidemic, perpetuating a state of urgency driven by notions of potentiality and futurity. This new tone of urgency in the era of "treatment as prevention" is perhaps most glaringly embodied in the policy rhetoric of UNAIDS in its 2011–2015 strategy for "Getting to Zero" [1] and its more recent "90-90-90" treatment target of getting 90 % of people living with HIV diagnosed, on treatment, and virally suppressed. Here the persistent sense of urgency not only gathers momentum around a concern for the improvement of life; but its affective force comes from the looming possibility of failure—that only politics, corruption, and economic interests could stand in the way of an "achievable" end to the HIV epidemic, an end that is now imaginable as firmly within our grasp. The impassioned rhetorical pleas of leading scientists at international AIDS conferences, although finding some echoes in activist responses, firmly places the possibility of and responsibility for such visions of "success" in the hands of scientific and public health experts. Therefore understanding how this perpetuation of such a state of urgency ushers in new policy regimes, animates new technological and technical investments, and ensures flows of funds (where it will go and how it will be accounted) is important for understanding how we have arrived at a moment in which the role of HIV activism and the utility of human rights-based approaches are increasingly drawn into question.

Larger global policy pronouncements that incite such states of urgency serve as an important interpretive backdrop in the stories I have told. However I have tended to avoid recounting a structuralist narrative of how the social reverberations of such

[1] The idea behind the rhetoric is about drastically reducing new infections and AIDS-related deaths by getting people on ARVs as soon as possible.

R. Lorway, *AIDS Activism, Science and Community Across Three Continents*, Social Aspects of HIV 1, DOI 10.1007/978-3-319-42199-5

important events dramatically transform local policy arenas, making them fall in line with global guidelines or "best practises." Instead I have focused on the smaller, more localized social practises and ordinary textures tying together members of diverse groupings of scientists, health officials and affected communities in particular times and places as they puzzle through, debate, and determine the knowledge that counts in program planning and implementation. Within the particular forms of evidentiary sovereignty I have tried to highlight across various geographies and temporalities, "evidence production" processes, including those in which I have directly participated, constitute an ever expanding territory that increasingly encompasses the far reaches of community practises, affective networks, and identities; but without ever fully subsuming these domains of sociality. In fact, they rely upon it to extend their authority. From this perspective of the more mundane makings and remakings of scientific knowledge hierarchies, then, we see more than just the clashes and collisions between experiential and expert knowledge, between affected communities and scientific and technical experts. We also view an increasing embroilment of scientists and activists together in the creation of *more precision-oriented approaches* to intervening and governing the health of populations.

In Canada, the credentialization of the HIV movement through the introduction and embrace of the community-based research capacity building initiative pivoted on the logic that "community knowledge"—on-the-ground practical wisdom accumulated over years of frontline practise—could refine epidemiological surveillance efforts to more swiftly detect and respond to changes in the HIV epidemic, bringing activists into closer relationships with academic researchers. Meanwhile, the treatment experiences and struggles of Nova Scotia HIV activists in the experimental era of ARVs, an era characterized by uncertainty and onerous treatment regiment, drew activists into the regulatory domains of clinical trials regulatory boards. In both instances, the co-evolution of activism and scientific knowledge was driven by attempts to thread the daily lived realities of highly affected communities through scientific knowledge procedures. And in so doing, activists became deeply and emotionally invested in scientific knowledge.[2]

In Mysore too, albeit from a more technocratic history of intervention, communities of male sex workers and men who have sex with men involved themselves in producing the knowledge that counted to intervention specialists. And through their encounters and engagements with the reigning geography of intervention, the priorities of these members of sexual minority rights organizations became entangled in various business logics and epidemiology notions. Although producing a terrain

[2] Allman (2015) makes an important point that not all social scientific research needs to be "community-based" as not all communities possess the specialized knowledge to take up certain forms of research. Nor do they necessarily want this knowledge. But the significance of this statement can be placed in historical context—why is it important to articulate this position at this moment in time? While I agree with the heart of Allman's argument, I also feel that the significance of the argument itself suggests that we have arrived at a moment in which (1) communities feel that they need to produce evidence to assert their credibility and political legitimacy and (2) the relationship of different groups of people, including marginalized and highly stigmatized groups, increasingly occupy a more intimate positionality within terrains of research knowledge production.

of local knowledges that reflect diverse, ambiguous, partial and hybrid understandings of scientific knowledge, evidence matter to these social movement actors because it plays a crucial role in how they steer the course between financial and health security in their everyday lives. The frustration that erupted following the transition of Avahan to the public system reveals how affectively invested in evidentiary regimes these communities have become, such that their politicized objections raised around the tyranny of form filling goes beyond a concern for the avalanche of paper work and the state's attempt to wrestle "community mobilization" under its dominion. These communities are also deeply concerned by the quality and accuracy of the evidence generated by the newly standardized system that inadvertently fosters fake form filling practises.

And thirdly, Nairobi sex workers, who have long engaged with the bio-experimental practises and projects of Kenyan and Canadian scientists, were forced to confront new power arrangements with the formation of a South-to-South partnership. Indian and Kenyan scientists, although contending with initial postcolonial tensions, quickly found synergy between Avahan's geography of intervention and the longer history of immunological studies. With respect to sex work, the partnership originally ignited hope that their participation would more meaningfully and forcefully position the interests of sex workers in HIV decision making arenas, like they imagined it had for their Indian peers. However it soon became apparent that their participation in enumerative procedures only increased the external regulation of their organization activities through the re-assertion of questionable denominators and coverage targets that ranked their organization's productivity against other CBOs throughout Kenya. Dissent broke out of the bio-experimental governance of their sexual health, as the very ground from which their social movement emerged becomes inflamed, erupting into less publically visible but highly emotionally charged rebellions against the clinic and the coercive modes of tracking such as biometric protocols. At the same time, sex workers' willingness and enthusiasm to participate in clinical trials reflected their political commitment to exploring bio-experimental futures with clinical scientists.

My retelling of these stories attempts to show how evidentiary sovereignty matters and materializes in particular locales and specific temporalities. Cutting across these three case studies, it can be seen how "community health promotion" (and it variations such as empowerment and community mobilization) and an array of techniques for defining key populations (whether through the terms of business science, demography, epidemiology or bio-experimental sampling) act as two different hands of the same bio-political sovereign, working in tandem to guide community participation into the fold of technocratic governance. This Foucauldian perspective co-implicates communities and scientists in the remaking of epistemological hierarchies that have brought us to this technocratic moment, a social process that has been brewing since the very early years in particular factions of HIV activism, and which has transformed itself around successive scientific advances.

But this is only part of the story of evidentiary sovereignty. It is also vital to recognize that the various unfoldings of specialized knowledge regimes that govern responses across time and space has neither fully co-opted nor domesticated nor contained HIV activism. In fact, the way activists and affected communities interpret and utilize scientific knowledge exceeds the original expectations and aims of the experts that design interventions. As we attend to the complex life history of evidence production processes, we see how communities become increasingly literate in the workings of power, and cultivate their own strategies to maximize their interests in policy making arena across various geographic and temporal scales. Thus these case studies enable us to see the ontology of "evidence" as it lived out in the real world of intervention practises—as complex assemblages of universalistic forms of expert knowledge; local experiences, observations, and reasonings—and the transnational affective ties that hold these assemblages together while outwardly extending their influence. It is also important to recognize that for highly affected communities the standardizing effects of enumerative regimes increasingly shape similarly experiences and struggles around which transnational activist alliances and networks rally their members, as well as the researchers and policy makers who are sympathetic to their cause.

We certainly can applaud the acuity of activists and communities to "understand the relevant science" in order to assert their political credibility and moral authority, as Cindy Patton (2002:20) has remarked with respect to ACT UP members. But the point here is not to assess how well lay people and activists "know" their science. For certain, HIV activists emerging among communities of people who have little formal education or training in scientific thought may hold ideas that might be judged as simply erroneous by the standards of conventional science. Moreover, we have entered an era in which increasingly complex, specialized, and inaccessible HIV science is being put into the realm of practise. However, the force of activism in relation to contemporary HIV science is best realized in its ability to affect the very social "systems and the processes through which science is produced" (Patton 2002:19). What I find most remarkable is how contemporary forms of activism and community engagements are able to make science relevant and practical in the daily life of programs and interventions, in ways that experts might not expect.

At the same time we should not overlook the growing anxieties, fears and moral outrage expressed by activists with respect to this technocratic era in favour of a perspective often advanced in social studies of science and technology—that is, a "horizontal view" that would flatten out the relevance of how the political economy of global health science reinforces deep inequalities between low, mid, and high income countries.[3] For instance, the biometric tracking of criminalized groups in Kenya, which would be politically unacceptable in Western nations, is tied to the growing tendency to offshore clinical trials in low and middle income countries (Petryna 2009), a part of the global health scientific industry that clearly serves the marketing and professional interests of Western researchers. Moreover, the increasing trend toward precision-oriented approaches (mapping, biometrics, tracking forms, biological specimen, and genotyping), driven by the logic of verification and accountability, hold rather disturbing implications for how techniques of measure-

[3] Johann Crane's compelling ethnography seeks a rapprochement between science studies and political economy in what she terms "critical science studies".

ment and surveillance have begun (and may in the future) articulate with the intensified criminalization of highly affected groups in Canada, India, and Kenya. My seemingly particularistic rendering of activism, science and sovereignty is not intended to ignore these political economic implications. Rather my attempt has been to point to the vital (although often uncomfortable) spaces in which the critical social sciences can directly engage with the HIV activist agenda of affecting science.

References

Allman, D. (2015). Community centrality and social science research. *Anthropology & Medicine*, *22*(3), 1–17.

Patton, C. (2002). *Globalizing aids*. Minneapolis: University of Minnesota Press.

Petryna, A. (2009). *When experiments travel: Clinical trials and the global search for human subjects*. Princeton: Princeton University Press.

MIX
Papier aus verantwortungsvollen Quellen
Paper from responsible sources
FSC® C105338

If you have any concerns about our products,
you can contact us on
ProductSafety@springernature.com

In case Publisher is established outside the EU,
the EU authorized representative is:
Springer Nature Customer Service Center GmbH
Europaplatz 3, 69115 Heidelberg, Germany

Printed by Libri Plureos GmbH
in Hamburg, Germany